A Senior  le
to a
Happy Sex Life

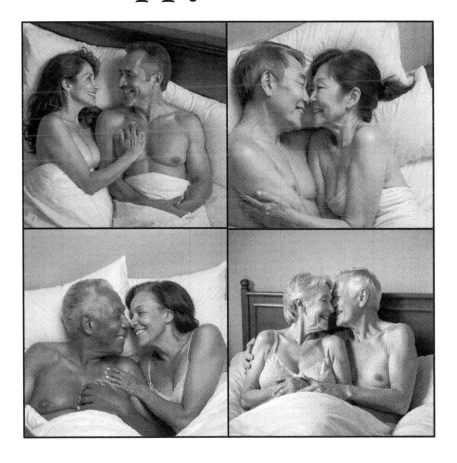

Enhancing Communication, Emotional Bonding, Intimacy, and Adaptation

by
Dr. Robert J. Walker

A Senior Citizen Guide to a Happy Sex Life

by

Dr. Robert J. Walker

Amazon.com inc.
P.O. Box 81226
Seattle, WA 98108-1226
https://kdp.amazon.com
1-888-280-4331

ISBN: 9798329695557

Cover Photos created using OpenArt AI.

Contents

Dedication

The classification of "senior citizen" can vary depending on context, region, and organization. In some contexts or organizations, a 55-year-old individual might be considered a senior or eligible for certain benefits:

1. **AARP Membership**: In the United States, individuals can join AARP (formerly known as the American Association of Retired Persons) at age 50.
2. **Senior Living Communities**: Some senior living communities and retirement homes have entry ages starting at 55.
3. **Discounts**: Certain businesses or organizations might offer senior discounts starting at age 55.
4. **Early Retirement**: Some pension plans and retirement systems allow for early retirement starting at 55.

Generally, the term "senior citizen" is more commonly associated with individuals who are 65 years old or older, primarily due to retirement age and eligibility for senior-specific benefits and services such as Social Security and Medicare in the United States.

Whether you are between the ages of 55 to 64, and not yet ready to embrace the label of "senior citizen", or if you are 65 or older, *A Senior Citizen Guide to a Happy Sex Life* is dedicated to helping you to enhance your sexual pleasure at any age.

Introduction

Welcome to *A Senior Citizen Guide to a Happy Sex Life*, where age is merely a number and pleasure knows no bounds. In these pages, you will embark on a journey challenging the stereotypes and misconceptions surrounding intimacy in the later years of life. With candid advice, insightful reflections, and practical tips, this guide is a roadmap to rediscovering the joys of physical connection, intimacy, and fulfillment at every stage of life. Whether you're reigniting the flames of passion with a long-time partner or navigating a new relationship, let's embark together on a liberating exploration of love, desire, and the endless possibilities of a fulfilling sex life in our golden years.

Having sexual desires in your senior years doesn't mean that you are a dirty old man or a dirty old woman. It just means that you are human. Therefore, if your children or grandchildren have a problem with it—tell them, "Get over it and mind your own business!"

As we journey through life, our understanding and experience of sexuality evolve, and that doesn't change as we age. Good sex for senior citizens is a topic often overlooked or dismissed, yet it's a vital aspect of well-being and quality of life for many older adults. In this guide, we'll explore the nuances and benefits of sexual intimacy in the later years, debunking myths, addressing challenges, and highlighting the joys and pleasures that come with age. From physical health to emotional connection, it's vital to understand the importance of a fulfilling sexual relationship in our senior years and how to maintain it with vitality and vigor.

As we age, our perception of sex and intimacy often undergoes significant transformations. Contrary to common misconceptions, the desire for sexual expression doesn't diminish with age; rather, it adapts, evolving into a rich tapestry of emotional connection, physical pleasure, and profound intimacy. Exploring the realm of good sex for those of us in our senior years unveils a landscape where experience, wisdom, and mutual respect intertwine to create deeply fulfilling relationships. In this guide, we delve into the intricacies of sexual well-being among us older adults, celebrating the diverse expressions of love and passion that continue to thrive throughout our golden years.

The Desire For Connection and Physical Pleasure

Navigating the landscape of sexual intimacy in the later stages of life unveils a realm rich with nuance, depth, and resilience. Contrary to societal stereotypes, the desire for connection and physical pleasure doesn't wane as one grows older; rather, it evolves, shaped by a lifetime of experiences, wisdom, and emotional maturity.

In *A Senior Citizen Guide to a Happy Sex Life*, we will embark on a journey to explore the concept of good sex for senior citizens—a journey marked by profound intimacy, renewed passion, and a celebration of the diverse expressions of love that transcend age. From debunking myths to embracing the unique joys and challenges that come with maturity, we uncover the essential ingredients for maintaining a vibrant and fulfilling sexual relationship in the later chapters of life.

Debunking Misconceptions

While society often overlooks or underestimates the vitality of sexual expression in later years, the reality for many senior citizens is far richer and more nuanced than stereotypes suggest. In this guide, we will embark on an exploration of the intricacies of good sex for senior citizens, delving into the tapestry of emotions, desires, and experiences that shape intimate relationships in our golden years. From debunking misconceptions to celebrating the resilience and wisdom that age brings, we uncover the essence of sexual well-being among us older adults, embracing a narrative that honors the beauty and complexity of love and desire regardless of age.

For senior citizens, the notion of good sex transcends mere physical gratification; it encompasses a rich array of emotional connections, mutual respect, and shared intimacy. Contrary to prevailing myths that portray aging as a decline in sexual desires, as an older adult, you may have found yourself embracing a newfound sense of liberation and authenticity in your sexual life. Freed from the pressures of reproduction and societal expectations, as a senior, you may have already discovered a deeper appreciation for the pleasures of the flesh, guided by a lifetime of experience and self-discovery. However, navigating the terrain of sexual intimacy in the later years comes with its own set of challenges and considerations. Physical changes, such as decreased libido, erectile dysfunction, or menopausal symptoms, can pose obstacles to sexual satisfaction. Moreover, societal taboos and ageist attitudes may contribute to feelings of shame or inadequacy, inhibiting you or your mate from fully embracing your sexuality. Yet, amidst these challenges lies an opportunity for growth, resilience, and reimagining what it means to experience pleasure and intimacy in our later years.

A Senior Citizen Guide to a Happy Sex Life seeks to debunk the myths and misconceptions surrounding sex and aging, shining a light on the diverse expressions of desire and connection that flourish among senior citizens. Through candid discussions and expert insights, we delve into the physical, emotional, and relational aspects of sexual well-being in later life. From the importance of communication and consent to the role of intimacy-enhancing techniques and therapies, we uncover the essential ingredients for fostering a vibrant and fulfilling sexual relationship.

Embracing a Holistic Approach to Sexual Health

Moreover, we celebrate the resilience and wisdom that come with age, recognizing that the journey toward sexual fulfillment is as unique and varied as the individuals who embark upon it. By embracing a holistic approach to sexual health—one that acknowledges the interconnectedness of mind, body, and spirit—we honor the innate human desire for intimacy and connection, regardless of age or stage in life. In doing so, we affirm the inherent dignity and worth of each of us as senior citizens.

Each chapter of this guide provides ideas with specific tips and insights for maintaining a healthy and satisfying sex life. This guide also highlights the importance of communication, emotional bonding, intimacy, and adaptation in the development of a happy sex life.

A final point in this Introduction is the fact that the key ingredient to having a happy fulfilling sex life with your partner is honest and open communication. You will hear this fact echoed throughout the pages of this guide. I know at times; honest and open communication tends to be a hard thing for men to do. Especially if it could be that the man may be the one who has a problem in the sexual department. However, without open and honest communication, the recommendations given in this guide will not be successful.

May this guide serve as a tool to help you reclaim your right to pleasure, passion, and a love that knows no bounds.

Chapter 1: Good Sex for Senior Citizens

Sexuality is a natural and integral part of the human experience, yet societal stigmas often cast a shadow over the sexual lives of senior citizens. As we age, we may encounter various challenges and barriers to maintaining a fulfilling and satisfying sex life. However, it's essential to recognize that age should not be a deterrent to intimacy and sexual wellness.

Sexuality is a fundamental aspect of human existence, yet discussions about sex and aging often skirt around the lived experiences of senior citizens. In our youth-centric culture, the sexual desires and needs of older adults are often sidelined, perpetuating harmful stereotypes and societal stigmas. However, it's crucial to challenge these misconceptions and redefine what constitutes good sex for senior citizens. By dismantling ageist attitudes and promoting a more inclusive understanding of sexuality in later life, we can embrace our sexual vitality and enjoy fulfilling intimate relationships.

Sexuality and intimacy are vital aspects of the human experience, contributing significantly to emotional, psychological, and physical well-being. As we age, societal perceptions often mistakenly assume that sexual activity and desire diminish or become irrelevant. However, good sex for senior citizens remains not only possible but also beneficial, fostering connection, enhancing quality of life, and promoting overall health.

Good sex for senior citizens is a multifaceted concept that encompasses physical health, emotional well-being, and relational satisfaction. By challenging stereotypes, addressing health-related challenges, and fostering open communication, as seniors we can enjoy fulfilling and meaningful sexual experiences. Embracing sexuality in later life not only enhances individual well-being but also enriches relationships, promoting a holistic approach to aging gracefully and joyfully.

Importance of Sexual Health in Later Life

As societies evolve and lifespans lengthen, the narrative surrounding aging has undergone a transformation. No longer is it solely about decline and limitation, but increasingly about vitality and well-being, even in later years.

Within this shift, discussions about sexual health for senior citizens emerge as pivotal. Contrary to stereotypes, sexual health in later life holds significant importance for physical, emotional, and relational well-being. There are myriad reasons why nurturing sexual health among senior citizens is crucial, including the impact that sexual health has on physical health, emotional satisfaction, and the dynamics of relationships.

Physical Health: Sexual activity, even in later life, is associated with a plethora of physical health benefits. Studies have shown that regular sexual activity can lower blood pressure, reduce the risk of heart disease, and strengthen the immune system. Engaging in sexual activity increases blood flow, leading to improved circulation, and can alleviate chronic pain through the release of endorphins. Moreover, it has been linked to better sleep quality, which is crucial for overall health and cognitive function. Therefore, a healthy sex life in later life directly contributes to the holistic well-being of senior citizens.

Emotional Satisfaction: Sexuality is an integral aspect of human identity, influencing emotional fulfillment throughout the lifespan. For senior citizens, maintaining a healthy sex life can foster a sense of vitality and self-esteem. It provides avenues for self-expression, intimacy, and pleasure, enhancing overall life satisfaction. Research suggests that individuals who remain sexually active in later life are more content and happier. Additionally, sexual activity releases oxytocin and dopamine, neurotransmitters associated with bonding and pleasure, promoting emotional resilience and reducing stress. Thus, prioritizing sexual health for senior citizens is essential for nurturing emotional well-being and resilience.

Engaging in sexual activity later in life is also associated with a myriad of physical health benefits. Regular sexual activity has been linked to improved cardiovascular health, including lower blood pressure and reduced risk of heart disease. The physical exertion involved in sexual activity can also contribute to increased flexibility, muscle tone, and overall physical fitness. Moreover, the release of endorphins during sexual arousal can alleviate chronic pain and promote relaxation, leading to improved sleep quality. Thus, prioritizing your sexual health can directly contribute to your physical well-being, enhancing vitality and longevity.

Sexuality is an integral aspect of human identity and plays a significant role in emotional satisfaction throughout the lifespan. As senior citizens, maintaining a healthy sexual life can contribute to our sense of vitality, self-esteem, and overall life satisfaction. Sexual intimacy provides avenues for self-expression, connection, and pleasure, fostering a deeper sense of intimacy and emotional fulfillment. Research has shown that individuals who remain sexually active in later life report higher levels of happiness and lower rates of depression. Thus, nurturing sexual health among senior citizens is essential for promoting emotional well-being and resilience in the face of life's challenges.

Relationship Dynamics: Sexual intimacy plays a pivotal role in the dynamics of romantic relationships, regardless of age. For those of us who are senior citizens, maintaining a satisfying sexual connection with our partner can strengthen bonds, foster mutual understanding, and reignite passion.

Open communication about sexual needs and desires becomes increasingly important as we age, facilitating intimacy and deepening emotional connection. Moreover, shared sexual experiences can reignite passion, rekindle romance, and enhance relationship satisfaction. Shared sexual experiences can also contribute to a sense of closeness and companionship. By prioritizing sexual health in later life, we can nurture fulfilling and enduring relationships, thus promoting overall relational well-being.

Challenges and Considerations: Despite the importance of sexual health in later life, numerous challenges and considerations exist. Physical limitations, such as chronic illness or mobility issues, may impact sexual function and desire. Additionally, societal attitudes and stereotypes about aging and sexuality can create barriers to open discussion and access to resources.

As society progresses and attitudes toward aging evolve, the importance of sexual health in later life emerges as a crucial aspect of overall well-being for those of us who are senior citizens. Contrary to outdated stereotypes portraying aging as a time of decline and disengagement from intimacy, research, has highlighted the significance of maintaining a fulfilling sexual life well into old age.

As seniors, embracing sexual health in later life is essential for our holistic well-being. From physical health benefits to emotional satisfaction and relationship dynamics, sexual activity plays a multifaceted role in enhancing quality of life. By prioritizing sexual health, as senior citizens, we can maintain vitality, strengthen relationships, and experience greater emotional fulfillment as we age. Addressing the challenges and fostering supportive environments are essential steps towards ensuring that as senior citizens we can fully embrace and enjoy our sexual well-being.

Overcoming Societal Stigmas

As society progresses, discussions around sexuality have become more inclusive, yet we as senior citizens are often overlooked in these conversations. The stigma surrounding the sexual lives of older adults persists, portraying us as devoid of desire or relevance in sexual matters. This stigma not only undermines our autonomy but also neglects the significant impact that healthy sexual expression can have on our overall well-being. To empower us in overcoming these societal stigmas and to embrace our sexuality, it's crucial for us to understand the roots of these misconceptions and explore strategies to overcome them.

In contemporary society, discussions about sex often revolve around the youth-centric narrative, leaving the sexual experiences and needs of senior citizens largely ignored or dismissed. This neglect stems from deeply ingrained societal stigmas surrounding aging and sexuality, which perpetuate harmful stereotypes and hinder open conversations about intimacy among older adults. However, it is imperative to challenge these stigmas and redefine what constitutes good sex for senior citizens.

Sexuality is an essential aspect of human well-being regardless of age. Therefore, let's take a few minutes to explore societal stigmas surrounding sex and aging, and examine the implications of these stigmas on senior citizens' sexual health and relationships, and propose strategies for overcoming these barriers so that you may have a more inclusive and fulfilling understanding of sexuality in later life.

Understanding Societal Stigmas

The stigmatization of senior citizens' sexuality stems primarily from three societal perceptions or biases:

1. **Ageism:** Ageist attitudes assume that older adults are no longer interested in or capable of sexual activity. This misconception overlooks the diversity of experiences and desires among us as seniors.
2. **Cultural Norms:** Cultural norms often emphasize youth and vitality in discussions about sexuality, marginalizing older adults who may not fit this idealized image.
3. **Media Representation:** Media depictions frequently reinforce stereotypes by portraying older adults as asexual or focusing solely on age-related sexual dysfunction.

Societal Stigmas Surrounding Sex and Aging: The intersection of sex and aging is often overshadowed by pervasive societal stigmas that contribute to the marginalization and invisibility of older adults' sexual experiences. These stigmas are rooted in ageism, a form of discrimination based on age, which portrays aging as a period of decline and loss rather than growth and fulfillment. Ageism also leads to the marginalization and invisibility of older adults' sexual experiences. Media representations and cultural narratives frequently reinforce stereotypes. Consequently, as older adults we are often portrayed as asexual beings, devoid of sexual desires or capabilities, perpetuating the misconception that sex is exclusively a young person's domain. This portrayal not only erases the sexual identities of older individuals but also contributes to our feelings of shame, embarrassment, or inadequacy when it comes to sex.

Moreover, societal attitudes towards aging and sexuality are heavily influenced by cultural norms and stereotypes, which reinforce gendered expectations and double standards. For instance, older men may be celebrated for their virility and sexual prowess, while older women are expected to have no sexual desires and to remain unfulfilled sexually. Older women are also often subjected to ageist and sexist remarks that diminish their sexual activity and desirability. These stereotypes not only undermine our confidence and self-esteem as older adults but also contribute to the loss of our sexual identities and experiences. These stereotypes reinforce inequalities and erode our confidence in our sexual selves. They also reinforce the notion that sex is exclusively for the young.

Implications on Senior Citizens' Sexual Health and Relationships: The perpetuation of societal stigmas surrounding sex and aging has profound implications for the sexual health and well-being of senior citizens. One significant consequence is the lack of access to comprehensive sexual education and healthcare services tailored to the needs of us as older adults. As a result, many older individuals may be unaware of age-related changes in sexual function and how to address them, leading to feelings of shame, embarrassment, or inadequacy.

Furthermore, the stigma surrounding sex and aging can negatively impact our intimate relationships and social interactions. Fear of judgment or rejection may prevent us from openly discussing our sexual desires and preferences with our partner, leading to communication barriers and relationship strain. Additionally, as older adults, we may face societal barriers to forming a new romantic relationship or engaging in a casual sexual encounter due to ageist assumptions about sexuality and attractiveness.

Strategies for Overcoming Societal Stigmas

Sexuality is a fundamental aspect of human nature that transcends age, yet societal stigmas often overshadow the sexual experiences and desires of senior citizens. Empowering yourself to embrace your sexuality involves challenging stereotypes and fostering a more supportive environment for yourself and your partner. Here are some suggestions on ways to overcome stigmas about aging and sexuality:

1. Education and Awareness
Educational initiatives aimed at dispelling your own myths about aging and sexuality are essential. In addition to this guide, you can receive accurate information through workshops, seminars, and resources designed to help you understand that sexual desire and enjoyment can persist throughout life. Reliable sources of information, such as books, articles, or educational workshops, can provide valuable insights into maintaining sexual wellness in

later life. Speak to your doctor or a trusted healthcare service provider if you feel you have unique concerns.

By educating yourself and your partner about the realities of aging and sexuality, you will both gain a better understanding of your sexual health and well-being. This can also dispel myths and misconceptions and empower you to make informed decisions about your sexual lives.

2. Encourage Open Dialogue
Open communication with your partner is essential for overcoming barriers and for fostering intimacy. You should initiate honest and non-judgmental conversations about your sexual desires, preferences, and concerns. Creating a safe and supportive space for dialogue can help you and your partner navigate age-related changes in sexual function and maintain a fulfilling sex life.

If you are single, you should seek out social connections and community support to combat feelings of isolation and loneliness. Participating in group activities, joining senior centers or clubs, or engaging in online forums can provide opportunities for connection and companionship. Building strong social networks can also help challenge ageist attitudes and promote positive representations of sexuality in your senior years.

3. Seek Positive Role Models
Researching stories of older adults who maintain fulfilling sexual relationships can challenge stereotypes and inspire you to embrace your sexuality without shame. Positive role models provide visibility and validation for your sexual desires.

4. Address Healthcare Needs
Seek healthcare providers who are trained to address the sexual health concerns of older adults sensitively and comprehensively. This includes discussing age-related changes in sexual function, providing appropriate medical interventions, and offering counseling or referrals as needed.

5. Self-Care and Exploration
Taking care of your physical and emotional well-being is crucial for maintaining sexual vitality as a senior citizen. You must prioritize self-care practices such as regular exercise, healthy eating, and adequate sleep, which

can positively impact overall health and sexual function. Additionally, managing stress and practicing relaxation techniques can help reduce anxiety and enhance sexual pleasure.

Exploring new forms of intimacy and sexual expression can also be empowering. You can experiment with sensual massage, erotic literature, or erotic art to reignite passion and creativity in your intimate relationship. Embracing a mindset of curiosity and exploration can lead to new discoveries and deeper connections with yourself and your partner.

6. Advocate for Your Sexual Needs
Advocate with your partner for your own sexual health needs and preferences is crucial. Asserting your autonomy and making informed decisions about your sexual desires fosters a sense of empowerment and dignity.

Conclusion:
Overcoming your own societal stigmas concerning good sex for senior citizens requires a multifaceted approach that addresses the intersecting factors of ageism, sexism, and cultural norms. It requires a proactive approach that encompasses education, communication, and self-care. By challenging your own ageist beliefs, fostering open dialogue, and prioritizing sexual wellness, you can reclaim your sexual activity and enjoy fulfilling intimate relationships with your partner.

Embracing your sexual vitality will serve as a testament to your resilience and strength. It will enable you to transcend age and societal expectations. By education and awareness, and fostering inclusive healthcare and social environments, you can embrace your sexual identity and enjoy a fulfilling intimate relationship with your partner.

The quest for good sex knows no age limits, and it is imperative that you recognize and celebrate the inherent value of sexuality throughout the aging process. Embracing sexual vitality is a testament to the resilience and vitality of the human spirit, transcending age and societal expectations.

Overcoming societal stigmas concerning good sex for senior citizens requires a proactive approach that encompasses education, communication, and self-care. By challenging your own ageist beliefs, fostering open dialogue, and prioritizing sexual wellness, you can reclaim your sexual agency and enjoy a fulfilling intimate relationship.

Removing your own stigmas surrounding senior citizens' sexuality requires a collective effort to educate yourself on your misconceptions about aging and sexuality. You must be willing to reexamine the religious and cultural taboos you grew up with related to sex. As a senior citizen, you must reprogram your thoughts to recognize that you have the right to enjoy fulfilling and satisfying sexual experiences regardless of your age.

By embracing your sexuality as a natural and valuable aspect of your life, you will improve your overall well-being, strengthen your relationship, and enhance the quality of your life. Embracing a more inclusive and respectful attitude towards your sexuality benefits you as an individual, your family, and your community alike, paving the way for a society where all individuals, regardless of age, feel validated, respected, and empowered in their sexual identities and expressions.

Ultimately, the quest for a happy sex life knows no age limits, and it's essential to recognize and celebrate the inherent value of sexuality throughout the aging process. Once you and your partner allow yourselves to overcome your own or societal stigmas surrounding good sex in your senior years and reclaim your sexual activity, you will be able to cultivate a healthy and vibrant intimate life together. It's time for us as senior citizens to assert our rights to sexual fulfillment and live our lives with dignity and joy.

Chapter 2: Understanding the Aging Body

A happy sex life in your senior years involves recognizing and adapting to the natural changes that come with aging. As we age, our bodies undergo various physical transformations that can affect sexual health and activity. Understanding these changes is crucial for maintaining a fulfilling sex life. Understanding the aging body and its impact on sexual health enables us to adapt and find new ways to enjoy a satisfying sex life. Communication, medical support, emotional connection, and healthy lifestyle choices can lead to continued sexual fulfillment in later years.

Physical Changes in Women

As women age, their bodies undergo numerous physical transformations that can influence their sexual health and experiences. Understanding these changes is essential for maintaining a fulfilling and satisfying sex life during the senior years. Although there are physical changes that aging women experience, having insight into how to adapt and embrace these changes is key to better sexual health and intimacy:

1. Hormonal Changes and Menopause
One of the most significant changes that occur in a woman's body with age is menopause. This natural biological process marks the end of menstrual cycles and is typically diagnosed after 12 consecutive months without a period. Menopause usually occurs between the ages of 45 and 55, but it can vary.

According to the National Menopause Society (NMS), during menopause, some women feel more relaxed and enjoy sex more frequently because they do not have to worry about getting pregnant. Also, the children are grown and out of the home. Therefore, more time is available to enjoy sex and to have spontaneous sex without the responsibilities of raising children or the fear that one of your children may walk by your bedroom and hear the two of you making love. However, for many women, due to a major drop in estrogen, the classic menopause symptoms of hot flashes, night sweats, exhaustion, mood swings, the loss of bladder control, and urinary tract infections take away from their sexual desires. Treatment for these symptoms is often necessary in order to get your groove back.

2. Decline in Estrogen Levels

Estrogen is a hormone responsible for regulating the menstrual cycle and maintaining vaginal health. Estrogen helps keep the lining of the vagina elastic, flexible and moisturized. Estrogen decreases significantly during menopause. This decline can lead to several changes, including vaginal dryness, thinning of the vaginal walls, and decreased vaginal elasticity. These changes can cause discomfort or pain during intercourse, known as dyspareunia, and may reduce overall sexual desire.

3. Urogenital Health and Vaginal Atrophy

Vaginal dryness is common as a woman age. Reduced estrogen levels can result in less natural lubrication, making the vaginal tissues drier and more fragile. This can lead to discomfort or pain during sexual activity. Vaginal atrophy is the thinning and inflammation of the vaginal walls. Vaginal atrophy can cause irritation and a decrease in vaginal elasticity, impacting sexual pleasure.

4. Decreased Libido

Hormonal fluctuations, along with other factors like stress, health conditions, and medications, can lead to a decrease in sexual desire. It's important to recognize that changes in libido are natural and can be addressed through various means.

5. Changes in Orgasmic Response

Aging can affect the intensity and frequency of orgasms. Women might experience weaker or less frequent orgasms due to changes in blood flow and nerve sensitivity in the genital area.

Female Adaptations and Strategies for Maintaining a Healthy Sex Life

1. Open Communication

Discussing sexual needs, preferences, and any discomforts with your partner is crucial. Honest communication can help in finding mutually satisfying solutions and maintaining intimacy. Be open with your partner about your menopausal symptoms.

2. Use of Lubricants:

Over-the-counter lubricants can alleviate vaginal dryness and make sexual activity more comfortable. Water-based or silicone-based lubricants are often recommended for their effectiveness and compatibility with most condoms and sex toys.

3. Vaginal Moisturizers and Estrogen Therapy:

Regular use of vaginal moisturizers can help maintain vaginal moisture and health. For some women, local estrogen therapy (available as creams, rings, or tablets) can effectively alleviate symptoms of vaginal atrophy.

4. Sexual Aids and Techniques:

Exploring different sexual positions and using sexual aids such as vibrators can enhance pleasure and accommodate physical changes. Finding comfortable and satisfying positions can make a significant difference.

5. Body Positivity and Self-Acceptance:

Embracing body changes and fostering a positive body image can significantly impact sexual satisfaction. Confidence in your body, regardless of age, enhances sexual experiences.

6. Emotional Intimacy:

Non-sexual forms of intimacy, such as cuddling, kissing, and sharing activities can strengthen emotional bonds with your partner. Emotional connection plays a vital role in a satisfying sex life.

7. Healthy Living:

Maintaining a healthy lifestyle through regular exercise, a balanced diet, and sufficient sleep contributes to overall well-being and can improve sexual health. Exercise, in particular, enhances blood flow and increases energy levels, positively affecting sexual desires and performance.

8. Stress Reduction:

Managing stress through mindfulness, meditation, or engaging in hobbies can positively impact sexual desire and performance. Reducing stress levels promotes relaxation and enhances sexual enjoyment.

9. Have More Sex:

Believe it or not, having more sex helps preserve vaginal tissue and the vagina from being irritated. Arousal boosts your tissue health by causing an increase in blood flow to your genitals. This is true even if you are satisfying yourself without your partner.

Conclusion:

Understanding the physical changes that occur in your body as you age is essential for adapting to and embracing these changes. By acknowledging and addressing hormonal shifts, vaginal health, and other factors, as a senior woman, you can maintain a fulfilling and satisfying sex life. Open communication, the use of lubricants and moisturizers, exploring sexual aids, and fostering emotional intimacy are all key strategies for enjoying good sex in your senior years. Embracing these changes with a positive mindset and healthy lifestyle choices can lead to continued sexual fulfillment and overall well-being.

Physical Changes in Men

Sexual health and intimacy remain important aspects of life, regardless of age. For a senior male, maintaining a satisfying sex life can positively impact emotional well-being, relationship quality, and overall life satisfaction. However, for men, the physical changes that come with aging can drastically affect sexual function. Understanding these changes is crucial for managing expectations and finding ways to adapt.

1. Changes in Hormone Levels
As men age, testosterone levels gradually decline. This hormonal change, often referred to as andropause, can impact sexual desire (libido) and performance. Testosterone is a key hormone in regulating libido and energy levels in men, so a decrease can lead to reduced sexual interest and stamina.

2. Erectile Dysfunction
Erectile dysfunction (ED) becomes more common with age. It can stem from various factors, including decreased blood flow, reduced testosterone levels, and underlying health conditions such as diabetes, hypertension, and cardiovascular diseases. ED can affect a man's confidence and ability to engage in sexual activity.

3. Reduced Sensitivity and Slower Arousal
Aging can lead to changes in nerve function, resulting in reduced sensitivity and slower arousal. Men may find it takes longer to become erect and achieve orgasm. Additionally, the firmness of erections may diminish, and the refractory period (the time needed to recover before becoming aroused again) may increase.

4. Physical Health Conditions
Chronic health conditions prevalent in us older men, such as diabetes, heart disease, and arthritis, can impact sexual function. These conditions can cause pain, fatigue, and mobility issues, all of which can affect sexual activity. Medications for these conditions can also have side effects that impact sexual performance.

5. Psychological Factors
Mental health plays a crucial role in sexual function. Anxiety, depression, and stress can negatively affect libido and performance. Concerns about aging and sexual adequacy can also lead to performance anxiety, further complicating sexual experiences.

Male Adaptations and Strategies for Maintaining a Healthy Sex Life

Despite these challenges, as a senior male, you can still enjoy a fulfilling sex life. Here are some strategies to help manage the physical changes associated with aging:

1. **Open Communication**: Honest discussions with your partner about changes and expectations can reduce anxiety and improve intimacy. Understanding each other's needs and finding mutually satisfying ways to be intimate can strengthen your relationship.

2. **Healthy Lifestyle**: Maintaining a healthy diet, regular exercise, and managing chronic conditions can improve your overall health and sexual function. Exercise, in particular, boosts cardiovascular health, which is crucial for erectile function.

3. **Medical Consultation**: Consulting healthcare providers about sexual health is important. Treatments for ED, hormone therapy, and managing chronic conditions can enhance sexual function. Your doctor can also adjust your medications, such as blood pressure medication, that may be impacting your sexual performance.

4. **Focus on Intimacy**: Intimacy is more than just sexual intercourse. Emphasizing other forms of closeness, such as caressing, kissing, and massage, can maintain a strong connection with your partner and reduce performance pressure. Understand that it is okay if you do not have an orgasm. Your focus should be on pleasing your partner, not just simply on your own personal pleasure. Even if you, for whatever reason, are unable to get an erection during intimacy, it doesn't mean that you should deny your mate sexual pleasure.

5. **Sexual Aids and Therapies**: There are medical devices and therapies designed to assist with erectile function. Couples therapy or sex therapy can also be beneficial in addressing the emotional and psychological aspects of intimacy.

6. **Mindfulness and Relaxation Techniques**: Practicing mindfulness and relaxation techniques can reduce anxiety and improve sexual experiences. Techniques such as meditation, deep breathing, and yoga can enhance mental health and sexual performance.

Conclusion:
Aging brings about inevitable physical changes, but these changes do not spell the end of a satisfying sex life. By understanding these changes and adopting a proactive approach to health and communication, you as a senior man can continue to enjoy a meaningful and fulfilling sexual relationship. The key lies in embracing change, seeking appropriate medical advice, and focusing on the broader aspects of intimacy and connection.

Psychological and Emotional Changes

As we age, the landscape of intimacy and sexual health undergoes significant transformations. While societal stereotypes often dismiss the idea of seniors engaging in sexual activity, the reality is that many older adults continue to seek and enjoy intimate connections. Understanding the psychological and emotional changes that accompany aging can enhance the sexual well-being of us as senior citizens, fostering a more fulfilling and satisfying experience.

Psychological Changes

1. **Shift in Priorities and Expectations**:
   As we age, our priorities often shift from physical appearance and performance to emotional connection and companionship. As seniors, we often find that intimacy becomes less about physical prowess and more about the deep emotional bond shared with our partner.

2. **Body Image and Self-Esteem**:
   The natural aging process brings about changes in appearance, such as wrinkles, weight fluctuations, and reduced physical agility. These changes can impact self-esteem and body image, which in turn affects sexual confidence. However, as senior citizens, we must come to

accept and embrace these changes and focus on the emotional aspects of intimacy rather than physical perfection.

3. **Reduced Anxiety and Stress**:
   As older adults, we often experience a reduction in daily stressors such as career pressures and parenting responsibilities. This can lead to a more relaxed and stress-free approach to sex, allowing for greater enjoyment and connection with our partner.

4. **Cognitive and Emotional Resilience**:
   With age, we typically develop greater emotional resilience and cognitive flexibility. This can result in a more open and communicative approach to sexual health, allowing us to express our needs and desires more freely and thus fostering a deeper emotional connection.

Emotional Changes:

1. **Enhanced Emotional Intimacy**
   Emotional intimacy often becomes more significant as physical changes occur. We may prioritize emotional closeness, trust, and mutual respect over the physical aspects of sex. This shift can lead to a more profound and satisfying intimate connection.

2. **Acceptance and Authenticity**
   As older adults, we must learn to embrace our authentic selves, shedding societal pressures and unrealistic expectations. This acceptance can enhance emotional intimacy and will allow our partner to feel more comfortable being themselves and sharing their vulnerabilities.

3. **Renewed Focus on Pleasure**
   As the urgency of reproductive goals diminishes, the focus on sexual pleasure and experimentation can increase. You may explore new forms of intimacy and sexual expression, enhancing your overall sexual satisfaction.

4. **Navigating Loss and Grief**

As a senior, you may face the emotional challenges of losing a spouse or partner. The grief and loneliness that follow can impact your sexual health. However, forming new connections and allowing yourself to experience joy and pleasure again can be a vital part of the healing process.

Overcoming Barriers to Sexual Well-Being

Understanding and addressing the psychological and emotional changes you are experiencing as you get older is crucial in overcoming barriers to a healthy and fulfilling sex life. Here are some strategies to promote sexual well-being in later life:

1. **Open Communication**

Encourage open and honest communication with your partner about your needs, desires, and concerns. This can help alleviate anxieties and enhance emotional intimacy.

2. **Education and Awareness**:

Research accurate information about sexual health and aging can dispel myths and promote a positive attitude toward sex. Be open to discussing with your healthcare provider concerning your sexual health.

3. **Medical Support**:

Be open to addressing your medical conditions that affect your sexual health, such as erectile dysfunction or vaginal dryness, through appropriate treatments and therapies.

4. **Emotional Support**:

Counseling or therapy can be beneficial for dealing with emotional issues such as grief, anxiety, or depression. Mental health support can help navigate these challenges and improve your overall well-being.

5. **Adaptation and Flexibility**:
> Exploring different forms of intimacy and sexual expression can lead to greater satisfaction. This might include sensual touch, mutual masturbation, or other activities that foster closeness and pleasure.

Conclusion:

The psychological and emotional changes that accompany aging can significantly impact your sexual health and well-being. By understanding and addressing these changes, you can continue to enjoy a fulfilling and satisfying intimate relationship. Embracing emotional intimacy, open communication, and adaptability can lead to a vibrant and enriching sex life.

Chapter 3: Communication with Your Partner

Discussing sex can be a sensitive topic for senior citizens, but it's important for maintaining intimacy and a healthy relationship. By approaching the topic with care and mutual respect, as senior citizens, we can foster a deeper connection and enhance our intimate relationship.

Discussing Desires and Boundaries

As senior citizens, discussing desires and boundaries related to sex can be challenging but profoundly rewarding. As often stated in this guide, open communication is essential for a healthy and fulfilling intimate life. This chapter provides practical steps for conducting this important conversation with your partner:

1. Prepare Yourself Mentally and Emotionally
Before initiating the conversation, take some time to reflect on your own desires and boundaries. Understanding what you want and need is the first step toward communicating effectively.
- **Self-Reflection**: Consider what aspects of intimacy are most important to you. This might include emotional connection, physical comfort, frequency of sexual activity, and any new experiences you wish to explore.
- **Acknowledge Emotions**: It's normal to feel nervous or vulnerable when discussing such a personal topic. Recognize these feelings and remind yourself that open communication is key to a healthy relationship.

2. Choose the Right Time and Place
The setting for this conversation can significantly impact its success. Choose a time and place where both you and your partner feel relaxed and free from distractions.
- **Private and Comfortable**: Ensure the environment is private and comfortable for both of you. A relaxed setting can help ease any tension and promote open dialogue.

- **Unrushed**: Choose a time when you won't be interrupted or feel rushed. This allows both of you to express your thoughts and feelings fully.

3. Use Clear and Compassionate Communication

When discussing desires and boundaries, clarity and compassion are crucial. Approach the conversation with an open mind and a loving attitude.

- **Be Honest and Direct**: Clearly state your desires and boundaries without ambiguity. Use "I" statements to express your feelings and needs, such as "I feel" or "I need."
- **Listen Actively**: Pay attention to your partner's responses and validate their feelings. Active listening shows that you respect and value their perspective. Pay attention to your partner's body language.
- **Avoid Blame**: Focus on your own experiences and avoid blaming or criticizing your partner. This helps maintain a positive and constructive tone. Avoid slang sexual terms or overly clinical terms unless both partners are comfortable with them. Speak clearly and respectfully.
- **Regular Discussion**: Make discussions about sex a regular part of your relationship rather than a one-time conversation. Regularly discussing sex can help address issues as they arise and keep the intimacy alive.
- **Be Understanding**: Understand that discussing sex with your partner might be uncomfortable at first.
- **Have Patience**: Be patient with each other as you navigate these conversations, and approach the topic with kindness and understanding.

4. Discuss Physical Comfort and Health

Physical comfort and health are critical considerations for senior intimacy. Discuss any health concerns or physical limitations openly.

- **Health Considerations**: If you have health conditions that affect your sexual activity, share this information with your partner. Discuss ways to adapt and ensure both of you feel comfortable and safe.
- **Comfort and Safety**: Talk about what positions or activities feel comfortable for you. Establish mutual understanding and agreement on what works best for both of you.

- **Explore Alternatives**: If physical limitations are a concern, discuss alternative ways to maintain intimacy, such as snuggling, kissing, or non-sexual touch. Explore new ways to be intimate that are satisfying for both of you. Be open to trying new things. Exploring different forms of intimacy, such as massages, sensual touch, or even just spending quality time together, can enhance your connection.

5. Set Emotional Boundaries
Emotional readiness and comfort levels can vary widely. Setting emotional boundaries helps ensure that both partners feel secure and respected.
- **Emotional Needs**: Share your emotional needs and listen to your partner's. Discuss how to support each other emotionally and ensure that both of you feel loved and valued.
- **Respect Vulnerabilities**: Acknowledge any emotional vulnerabilities and agree on how to address them together. Building emotional trust can deepen your connection.

6. Explore New Possibilities Together
Intimacy in later life can be an opportunity to explore new experiences. Approach this exploration with curiosity and openness.
- **Be Open to Experimentation**: Discuss any new activities or experiences you'd like to try. Be open to your partner's suggestions and find common ground.
- **Maintain a Sense of Humor**: Approach new experiences with a lighthearted attitude. Laughing together can ease any awkwardness and enhance your bond.

7. Practice Safe Sex:
- **Protection:** Use protection to prevent sexually transmitted infections, especially if entering a new relationship.
- **Checkups**: Get regular sexual health checkups.

8. Ensure Mutual Consent:
- **Agree**: Ensure that all sexual activities are consensual and that both you and your mate feel comfortable and respected.

9. Seek Professional Guidance if Needed
If discussing desires and boundaries feels particularly challenging, consider seeking professional guidance.

- **Therapists and Counselors**: A therapist or counselor specializing in senior relationships can provide valuable support and facilitate effective communication.
- **Medical Professionals**: Consult healthcare providers for advice on managing health conditions that affect sexual activity. They can offer solutions and reassurance.

Conclusion:

Discussing desires and boundaries related to sex is a vital part of maintaining a healthy and fulfilling intimate life for those of us in our senior years. By preparing mentally and emotionally, choosing the right setting, communicating clearly and compassionately, and addressing physical and emotional needs, we can navigate these conversations successfully. Exploring new possibilities and seeking professional guidance, when necessary, can further enhance intimacy and strengthen the relationship. Embracing open dialogue about desires and boundaries paves the way for deeper connection, mutual respect, and lasting happiness.

Navigating New Dynamics

As senior citizens, navigating new dynamics related to sex can be approached thoughtfully and respectfully, considering the physical, emotional, and relational aspects involved. As we age, many aspects of our lives evolve, and our approach to a relationship and intimacy is no exception. Navigating the new dynamics of sex and intimacy can be both challenging and rewarding. Open and honest communication is key to ensuring that these challenges are addressed in a healthy and positive manner. Here are some points to consider when navigating these new dynamics:

Understanding the Changes
1. **Physical Changes**: Aging brings about changes in the body that can affect sexual function. A man may experience erectile dysfunction or reduced libido, while a woman might face issues like vaginal dryness or decreased arousal. Understanding these changes is the first step toward addressing them.

2. **Emotional and Psychological Factors**: Retirement, loss of a spouse, or changes in our finances or living conditions can impact our emotional state and, subsequently, our sexual desire and activity. Stress, anxiety, and depression are common among seniors and can influence sexual health.

3. **Health Conditions and Medications**: Chronic illnesses such as diabetes, heart disease, and arthritis, along with medications for these conditions, can affect sexual function. It's important to consider these factors when discussing sexual health.

4. **Be Open and Honest**: Share your feelings and concerns openly. Use "I" statements to express how you feel without blaming or accusing your mate. For example, "I've noticed some changes in my body, and I'm finding it difficult to enjoy sex as much as I used to."

5. **Listen Actively**: Allow your partner to share their thoughts and feelings without interruption. Active listening helps build empathy and understanding.

6. **Use Clear and Respectful Language**: Avoid euphemisms and be direct but gentle in your communication. Clear language helps in avoiding misunderstandings.

Conclusion:
Discussing sex as a senior citizen can be daunting, but it's a vital part of maintaining a healthy and fulfilling relationship. By understanding the changes presented in this section, by addressing these changes, and through honest and open communication, you can navigate the new dynamics of your sexual life with confidence, enjoyment, and health.

By understanding the changes, communicating openly, exploring solutions together, and maintaining a positive attitude, you and your partner can navigate the new dynamics of sex with confidence and grace. Remember, intimacy and connection are important at any age, and addressing these issues openly can lead to a deeper, more satisfying relationship.

Seeking Mutual Satisfaction

Seeking mutual satisfaction in a sexual relationship, regardless of age, involves open communication, understanding, and respect for each other's desires and boundaries. Here are some specific tips:

1. **Open Communication**: Talk openly and honestly with your partner about your desires, needs, and any concerns you may have. This creates a safe space for both of you to express yourselves without fear or judgment.

2. **Explore Together**: Take the time to explore each other's bodies and preferences. Experiment with different techniques, positions, and activities to find what brings both of you pleasure.

3. **Prioritize Foreplay**: As we age, we may find that we need more time and stimulation to become aroused. Spend ample time on foreplay to enhance arousal and intimacy.

4. **Be Patient**: Be patient and understanding with each other. It's normal for sexual function to change with age, and it may take longer to become aroused or achieve orgasm. Focus on enjoying the experience together rather than rushing to a specific outcome.

5. **Stay Healthy**: Maintaining overall health and well-being can contribute to sexual satisfaction. This includes physical checkups to include checking for sexually transmitted diseases (STDs), especially if you starting a new relationship. Staying physically active, eating a balanced diet, exercising, getting enough sleep, and managing any chronic health conditions you or your partner may have, are all vital to a healthy and happy sex life.

6. **Consider Medical Options**: If age-related changes are impacting sexual function, consider talking to a healthcare provider. There may be medical treatments or therapies available to address issues such as erectile dysfunction or vaginal dryness.

7. **Embrace Intimacy**: Remember that intimacy goes beyond sexual intercourse. Spend time cuddling, kissing, and expressing affection in non-sexual ways to deepen your emotional connection.

8. **Stay Positive**: A positive attitude can greatly enhance sexual satisfaction. Focus on the pleasure and joy that intimacy brings, rather than dwelling on any limitations or challenges.

9. **Educate Yourself**: Keep learning about sexuality and aging. There are many resources available, including books, workshops, and online forums, where you can learn from experts and share experiences with others in similar situations.

10. **Respect Boundaries**: Respect each other's boundaries and comfort levels. If either partner is not interested in sexual activity at a certain time, honor that decision without pressure or guilt.

Enhancing Intimacy and Satisfaction

As we age, our bodies and desires may change, but the need for intimacy and connection remains a fundamental aspect of human relationships. However, for many senior citizens, navigating sexual satisfaction can present unique challenges. Whether due to age-related changes in sexual function or societal taboos surrounding sexuality in older adults, seeking mutual satisfaction in sex requires understanding, communication, and a willingness to explore new possibilities. Some strategies for a senior citizen to enhance intimacy and satisfaction in their sexual relationship are:

Embrace Open Communication
Communication is key to any healthy relationship, and this holds true for sexual intimacy as well. You should feel empowered to openly discuss your desires, preferences, and any concerns you may have with your mate. This includes addressing physical changes, such as erectile dysfunction or vaginal dryness, as well as emotional needs and desires. By fostering open communication, you and your mate can better understand each other's needs and work together to find solutions that promote mutual satisfaction. It's important to approach these conversations with empathy, respect, and a willingness to listen without judgment.

Prioritize Physical and Emotional Connection

As previously stated, intimacy is about more than just sexual intercourse—it encompasses a range of physical and emotional experiences that deepen the bond between partners. It's about having a loving relationship throughout the day. You can enhance intimacy by prioritizing activities that promote physical and emotional connection, such as a walk in the park, opening the car door for your female companion, bringing flowers, hugging, a gentle kiss on the lips or cheek, and holding hands.

Engaging in regular physical affection can help maintain a sense of closeness and intimacy between partners, even if penetrative sex becomes less frequent or challenging due to age-related changes. By focusing on the emotional connection, you and your mate can cultivate a sense of intimacy that transcends the physical act of sex.

Explore New Techniques and Activities

As bodies age, sexual function may change, requiring a couple to explore new techniques and activities to maintain mutual satisfaction. This may involve experimenting with different positions, using lubricants to address vaginal dryness, or incorporating sex toys to enhance pleasure. You should approach sexual exploration with an open mind and a spirit of adventure. Trying new things together can reignite passion and excitement in the relationship while providing opportunities for mutual pleasure and satisfaction.

Prioritize Health and Well-Being

Maintaining overall health and well-being is essential for sexual satisfaction at any age. Certain lifestyle factors, such as smoking and excessive alcohol consumption, can negatively impact sexual function and satisfaction. By prioritizing healthy habits, you can support your sexual well-being and enhance your overall quality of life.

Conclusion:

By following these tips and maintaining open communication and mutual respect, you can continue to enjoy a fulfilling and satisfying sexual relationship. As previously stated, sexual intimacy is a natural and important aspect of human relationships, regardless of age. While you may encounter unique challenges in seeking mutual satisfaction, you can enhance intimacy and pleasure by prioritizing open communication, physical and emotional connections, exploration, and prioritizing health and well-being. By approaching intimacy with curiosity, compassion, and a willingness to adapt, you can continue to enjoy a fulfilling and satisfying sexual relationship well into your later years.

Chapter 4: Health Considerations

Health considerations can significantly affect the sex life of seniors in various ways: physical health issues, medications, chronic conditions, hormonal changes, body image concerns, and your mate's health are all factors that can affect your sex life. Overall, addressing these health considerations through open communication with healthcare providers, exploring treatment options, adapting sexual practices to accommodate physical limitations, and focusing on intimacy and emotional connection can help you maintain a fulfilling sex life.

Managing Chronic Conditions

As we age, we often face the reality of managing chronic conditions that can impact various aspects of our lives, including our sexual relationship. However, despite the challenges posed by health issues, intimacy remains an essential aspect of human connection regardless of age. Understanding how to navigate and manage chronic conditions within the context of a sexual relationship is crucial for maintaining physical, emotional, and relational well-being.

1. **Open Communication**: Effective communication serves as the cornerstone of any healthy relationship, especially when addressing sensitive topics such as sexual health. You should foster open and honest dialogues about your chronic conditions and how they affect your sexual intimacy. This includes discussing symptoms, limitations, concerns, and desires in a safe and non-judgmental environment.

2. **Educate Yourself**: Both partners should take the initiative to educate themselves about the specific chronic conditions they are managing and their potential impact on sexual health. This may involve consulting healthcare professionals, attending informational sessions, or researching reputable sources online. By understanding how you and your partner's conditions can affect sexual function and pleasure, you together can proactively explore strategies to mitigate challenges and enhance intimacy.

3. **Adaptation and Flexibility**: Living with chronic conditions often requires adaptation and flexibility in various aspects of life, including sexual activity. You may need to explore alternative sexual practices, positions, or techniques that accommodate physical limitations or discomfort. Additionally, being open to trying new approaches can foster creativity and deepen intimacy within the relationship.

4. **Prioritize Self-Care**: Maintaining overall health and well-being is essential for sustaining sexual vitality in later life. You should prioritize self-care practices such as regular exercise, balanced nutrition, adequate sleep, and stress management. Managing chronic conditions effectively often involves adhering to prescribed treatment plans, medications, and therapies, which can contribute to overall health and improve sexual function.

5. **Seek Professional Support**: It may be necessary for you and your mate to seek professional support from healthcare providers who specialize in sexual health or geriatric care. Healthcare professionals can offer personalized guidance, treatment options, and resources tailored to individual needs and preferences. This may include interventions such as medications, medical devices, counseling, or referrals to specialists as needed.

6. **Emotional Connection**: Emotional intimacy plays a significant role in sexual relationships, especially if you are navigating a chronic condition. Building emotional connections through trust, affection, and understanding can enhance sexual satisfaction and fulfillment. Engaging in activities that foster emotional closeness, such as shared hobbies, going on trips, playing board games, meaningful conversations, or non-sexual touch, can strengthen the bond between you and your partner and sustain intimacy over time.

7. **Supportive Environment**: Creating a supportive environment within the relationship is essential for managing chronic conditions and maintaining sexual well-being. This involves showing empathy, patience, and compassion towards each other's experiences and limitations. You and your mate should feel comfortable expressing your needs and desires without fear of judgment or rejection, fostering a sense of mutual respect and acceptance.

Conclusion:

Navigating sexual intimacy while managing chronic conditions can present unique challenges for a senior couple, but it's not insurmountable. By prioritizing open communication, education, adaptation, self-care, professional support, emotional connection, and a supportive environment, you and your mate can nurture intimacy and sustain a fulfilling sexual relationship well into later life. Ultimately, embracing these strategies can enrich the quality of life and strengthen the bond between the two of you, fostering a sense of connection, vitality, and joy in your shared journey.

Medications and Sexual Health

As we age, our bodies undergo numerous changes, and for many of us, managing health conditions with medications becomes a part of everyday life. While medications are essential for treating various ailments, it's important to recognize that they can also have unintended consequences, including effects on sexual health. For us seniors, maintaining a satisfying and fulfilling sex life can contribute significantly to our overall well-being and quality of life. Therefore, understanding how medications can impact sexual health is necessary.

The Link Between Medications and Sexual Health

Numerous medications prescribed to us senior citizens for conditions such as hypertension, diabetes, depression, and chronic pain can potentially affect our sexual function. These medications often work by altering hormone levels, neurotransmitter activity, or blood flow, inadvertently impacting sexual desire, arousal, and performance.

Common Medications and Their Effects

1. **Antidepressants**: Selective serotonin reuptake inhibitors (SSRIs) and tricyclic antidepressants, commonly prescribed for depression and anxiety, are notorious for causing sexual side effects such as decreased libido, delayed ejaculation, and erectile dysfunction.

2. **Antihypertensives**: Beta-blockers and diuretics used to manage high blood pressure can also interfere with sexual function by reducing

blood flow to the genitals, leading to erectile dysfunction in men and decreased vaginal lubrication in women.

3. **Antipsychotics**: Medications prescribed for conditions like schizophrenia and bipolar disorder may cause sexual side effects such as decreased libido, erectile dysfunction, and difficulty achieving orgasm.

4. **Hormone Therapy**: Hormone replacement therapy (HRT) and antiandrogen medications used to treat conditions like prostate cancer can lead to reduced libido, erectile dysfunction, and changes in sexual function due to alterations in hormone levels.

5. **Pain Medications**: Opioids and other pain relievers may cause sexual dysfunction by dulling sensation, reducing libido, and interfering with orgasm.

Addressing the Issue

1. **Open Communication**: You should feel comfortable discussing any sexual concerns with your healthcare provider. Honest communication enables healthcare professionals to assess the potential impact of medications on your sexual health and explore alternative treatment options.

2. **Medication Review**: You should be proactive in researching the medication your doctor prescribes to you. Periodic medication reviews are essential for identifying drugs that may be contributing to sexual dysfunction. Your healthcare provider can adjust dosages, switch medications, or prescribe additional treatments to alleviate sexual side effects while effectively managing your health condition.

3. **Lifestyle Modifications**: Adopting a healthy lifestyle can mitigate some of the sexual side effects of medications. Regular exercise, a balanced diet, adequate sleep, and stress management techniques can positively influence sexual function and overall well-being.

4. **Sexual Health Resources**: You and your mate can benefit from accessing resources such as sexual health counseling, support groups,

and educational materials tailored to your needs. These resources provide valuable information and support for addressing sexual concerns and maintaining intimacy in your relationship.

Conclusion:

While medications play a crucial role in managing health conditions among us seniors, it's essential to recognize their potential impact on sexual health. By fostering open communication, conducting medication reviews, and implementing lifestyle modifications, healthcare providers can help mitigate sexual side effects. Additionally, providing access to sexual health resources will empower you to address sexual concerns proactively and maintain a fulfilling sexual relationship as you age. Ultimately, a holistic approach to healthcare that considers both physical and emotional well-being is vital for preserving your sexual health and overall quality of life.

Maintaining Overall Health

Entering the golden years doesn't mean bidding farewell to a fulfilling sex life. In fact, prioritizing overall health can significantly enhance your sexual well-being. While aging brings physical changes, adopting a holistic approach to health can foster intimacy and vitality. Let's explore how you can maintain your overall health to improve your sexual life:

1. **Prioritize Physical Activity:** Regular exercise is a cornerstone of maintaining overall health, including sexual health. Engaging in physical activity boosts blood flow, strengthens muscles, and enhances flexibility, all vital for sexual function. You can choose low-impact exercises like walking, swimming, or yoga, tailored to your fitness level and mobility.

2. **Embrace a Balanced Diet:** A nutritious diet is essential for vitality and sexual health. You should focus on consuming whole foods rich in vitamins, minerals, and antioxidants. Incorporating fruits, vegetables, lean proteins, and whole grains can improve energy levels, mood, and libido. Additionally, staying hydrated is crucial for overall health and can alleviate issues like dryness. You should drink plenty of water.

3. **Maintain Mental Well-being:** Emotional and mental well-being play significant roles in sexual health. You should prioritize activities that reduce stress and promote relaxation, such as meditation, deep breathing exercises, or hobbies that you enjoy, such as growing a garden. Not only would a garden provide regular exercise, it is also an economical way to obtain fresh vegetables.

4. **Foster Communication:** Effective communication is key to maintaining intimacy and addressing sexual concerns. You should openly discuss your desires, concerns, and any physical changes with your mate and healthcare provider. Creating a supportive and understanding environment can strengthen your relationship with your mate and enhance sexual satisfaction for both of you.

5. **Prioritize Sleep:** Adequate sleep is crucial for overall health and vitality, including sexual function. You should aim for seven to nine hours of quality sleep per night. Establishing a relaxing bedtime routine, maintaining a comfortable sleep environment, and addressing any sleep disorders can improve energy levels and libido.

6. **Manage Chronic Conditions**: It is important to manage chronic health conditions that may impact sexual health. It may be necessary to manage these conditions through medication, lifestyle modifications, and regular medical checkups. Consulting with your healthcare provider can help you address concerns and explore treatment options without compromising your sexual well-being. Seeking therapy or support groups can also address underlying emotional concerns and foster a healthy relationship with your mate.

7. **Explore Sensuality:** Sexuality encompasses more than physical intercourse. You can explore sensuality through activities like cuddling, kissing, a shoulder rub, or extended foreplay. These acts foster intimacy and connection with your mate. Experimenting with new techniques and maintaining an open-minded attitude can reignite passion and pleasure.

8. **Practice Safer Sex:** Practicing safe sex is crucial, especially if you are engaging in a new relationship. Using condoms can prevent sexually transmitted infections (STIs) and promote sexual health. You should

also stay informed about STI prevention and testing. In prioritizing your well-being and that of your partner, it would be wise if both of you included STI testing as a part of your annual physical.

Conclusion:

As a senior citizen, you can enjoy a vibrant and fulfilling sex life by prioritizing your and your mate's overall health. By incorporating physical activity, maintaining a balanced diet, nurturing mental well-being, fostering communication, prioritizing sleep, managing chronic conditions, exploring sensuality, and practicing safe sex, you and your mate can experience intimacy, pleasure, and a happy sex life throughout your golden years. Embracing a holistic approach to health will empower you to live life to the fullest.

Chapter 5: Enhancing Intimacy

As we age, the nature of intimacy evolves. It becomes more about emotional connection, mutual understanding, and the deep bonds we share with our partner. Enhancing intimacy in later life can lead to more fulfilling sexual experiences and strengthen your relationship.

Importance of Emotional Connection

As we age, the dynamics of our relationships, including our intimate connection, undergo significant transformations. For senior citizen couples, maintaining a fulfilling and satisfying sexual life can sometimes present unique challenges. However, amidst the physical changes and societal stereotypes, there exists a profound truth: the importance of emotional connection in enhancing sexual intimacy knows no age limit.

Emotional connection forms the cornerstone of any healthy relationship, regardless of age. But for senior citizen couples, it takes on added significance in the context of their sexual lives. The physical aspects of intimacy may change over time due to factors such as health issues, medication, or hormonal changes. Yet, the emotional bond between partners can serve as a resilient foundation upon which to build and sustain a fulfilling sexual relationship.

One of the primary reasons why an emotional connection is crucial for senior citizen couples is its role in fostering trust and vulnerability. As we age, we may face insecurities about our bodies, performance, or desirability. In such moments, the presence of a supportive and understanding partner becomes invaluable. Emotional intimacy allows a couple to communicate openly about their fears, desires, and needs, creating a safe space where vulnerability is embraced rather than feared.

Moreover, emotional connection cultivates a deeper sense of intimacy beyond the physical realm. It involves being attuned to each other's feelings, thoughts, and experiences, thereby strengthening the bond between partners. This heightened sense of closeness can significantly enrich the sexual experience for you and your mate, transcending the mere act of physical intimacy and imbuing it with a profound sense of connection and mutual understanding.

Furthermore, emotional connection promotes empathy and compassion, essential qualities for navigating the complexities of aging and its impact on sexual health. As you and your mate empathize with each other's experiences and challenges, you can provide each other the support and reassurance needed to navigate these changes together. This shared journey fosters a sense of solidarity and mutual respect, deepening the emotional bond between the two of you and enhancing your sexual connection.

In addition to its role in enhancing sexual intimacy, emotional connection also contributes to overall relationship satisfaction and well-being for you and your mate. Research has consistently shown that couples who report higher levels of emotional intimacy tend to experience greater relationship satisfaction and longevity. By prioritizing emotional connection, you can cultivate a relationship that continues to flourish and evolve, even as you navigate the complexities of aging.

So, how can you and your mate nurture and strengthen your emotional connection to improve your sexual lives? Here are some suggestions:

1. First, as always, communication is key. Open and honest communication about desires, concerns, and expectations fosters a deeper understanding between your partner and you and promotes intimacy. Taking the time to listen attentively and empathize with each other's perspectives can go a long way in strengthening the emotional bond.

2. Secondly, prioritize quality time together. Engage in activities that foster connection and closeness, whether it's sharing hobbies, going for walks, or simply enjoying each other's company by watching a movie or a sporting event at home together. Building shared experiences strengthens the emotional connection and reinforces the bond between the two of you.

3. Lastly, don't underestimate the power of affection and small gestures of love. Simple acts such as holding hands, a kiss on the cheek, sending a text message to say, "I love you", cuddling, or expressing

appreciation for each other can reaffirm the emotional connection and keep the spark alive in the relationship.

The importance of emotional connection in enhancing your sex life cannot be overstated. By nurturing a deep and meaningful bond built on trust, empathy, and understanding, you can navigate the challenges of aging with grace and intimacy. Ultimately, it is this emotional connection that sustains and enriches your sexual relationship, allowing you to experience intimacy and fulfillment regardless of your age.

Conclusion:

In summary, emotional intimacy forms the foundation of a satisfying sexual relationship. It involves being open and honest with your partner, sharing your thoughts and feelings, and building a sense of trust and security. Here are three suggestions on how to deepen your emotional connection:

1. **Communicate Openly**: Share your feelings, desires, and concerns with your partner. Effective communication can help you understand each other's needs and expectations.

2. **Spend Quality Time Together**: Engage in activities you both enjoy. Whether it's a hobby, a walk, or a simple conversation over coffee, spending time together strengthens your bond.

3. **Show Appreciation**: Acknowledge and appreciate your partner's efforts and qualities. Simple gestures of love and gratitude can go a long way in enhancing intimacy. If you want to make love to your mate at the end of the day, you have to begin the romance first thing in the morning. Using kind words throughout the day such as, "Thank you." "I appreciate you." "You are wonderful!" "I love you."—will definitely ignite a spark of sexual desire by the time bedtime rolls around.

Non-Sexual Intimacy

As has been stated in the previous chapters—discussions about intimacy and sexual satisfaction, the focus often tends to be solely on the physical aspect.

However, an often-overlooked but crucial element in fostering a fulfilling sexual relationship in later years is non-sexual intimacy. In this section, we will explore the significance of non-sexual intimacy and how it contributes to improving your overall sexual well-being.

Understanding Non-Sexual Intimacy: Non-sexual intimacy encompasses a wide range of activities and behaviors that foster emotional closeness, trust, and connection between partners without necessarily involving sexual activity. As previously stated, this can include simple gestures such as holding hands, cuddling, hugging, kissing, or engaging in meaningful conversations. It's about the emotional bond that a couple share and the sense of closeness and security they derive from each other's presence.

As a senior couple, non-sexual intimacy plays a vital role in maintaining and enhancing your sexual life. Here are several reasons why:

1. **Emotional Connection**: As we age, the emotional connection between partners becomes increasingly important. Non-sexual intimacy allows you and your mate to strengthen your emotional bond, deepen your understanding of each other, and provide mutual support and comfort. This emotional closeness lays a solid foundation for a satisfying sexual relationship.

2. **Stress Reduction**: Aging comes with its share of stressors, including health concerns, financial worries, and lifestyle changes. Engaging in non-sexual intimacy, such as cuddling or spending quality time together, such as playing cards, dominoes, bowling, or even discussing this book together, can help alleviate stress and promote relaxation. When partners feel relaxed and at ease with each other, they are more likely to enjoy sexual intimacy.

3. **Communication and Trust**: Effective communication is key to any successful relationship, particularly in the realm of sexuality. Non-sexual intimacy encourages open and honest communication between you and your mate, allowing each of you to express your needs, desires, and concerns in a supportive environment. This fosters trust and understanding, paving the way for a fulfilling sexual relationship built on mutual respect and consent.

4. **Physical Well-being**: Non-sexual intimacy is not only beneficial for emotional and mental health but also for physical well-being. Activities such as gentle touch, hugs, kissing, and cuddling release oxytocin, a hormone associated with bonding and relaxation. These physical expressions of affection can promote feelings of arousal and desire, and enhance sexual stimulation.

5. **Rediscovering Intimacy**: As our bodies age and sexual function changes, we may need to explore new ways of experiencing intimacy. Non-sexual intimacy provides an opportunity for you and your partner to rediscover each other's bodies, preferences, and desires in a non-pressured and enjoyable manner. This exploration can reignite passion and excitement in the bedroom, leading to a more satisfying sexual experience.

Practical Tips for Incorporating Non-Sexual Intimacy:

- Set aside dedicated time for intimacy, free from distractions and obligations.
- Engage in activities that promote relaxation and connection, such as taking a leisurely walk together or enjoying a romantic dinner.
- Practice active listening and communicate openly about your feelings, desires, and boundaries.
- Be spontaneous and creative in expressing affection, whether through small gestures, such as bringing home your mate's favorite ice cream without him asking you, or bringing her a bouquet of flowers without it being a special day such as Valentine's Day or Mother's Day, or grand romantic gestures, such as buying her a nice necklace, or buying him a pair of slip-on tennis shoes without it being his birthday.
- Remember—intimacy is not solely about physical closeness but also about emotional connection and understanding.

Conclusion:

As a couple, seeking to keep or rekindle your sexual passion, you must always be mindful of the fact that intimacy isn't limited to sexual activity. Non-sexual intimacy can be just as fulfilling and can enhance your sexual relationship. Consider incorporating these elements into your relationship:

1. **Physical Affection**: Holding hands, hugging, and cuddling are important ways to express love and maintain physical closeness.
2. **Acts of Kindness**: Small acts of kindness, like making your partner's favorite meal or helping with a task, such as washing the dishes, show that you care and are attentive to their needs.
3. **Shared Activities**: Engage in activities that foster closeness, such as dancing, cooking together, or even reading to each other. These shared moments can deepen your connection.

In the journey of aging together, non-sexual intimacy serves as a cornerstone for maintaining a fulfilling and satisfying sexual relationship. By prioritizing emotional connection, communication, and mutual support, you can enhance the bond and reignite passion and intimacy regardless of your age. Embracing the importance of non-sexual intimacy will lead to a richer, more vibrant, and more satisfying sexual life for you and your mate.

Rediscovering Each Other

As we age, the dynamics of our relationship often shift, influenced by factors such as health issues, retirement, and an empty nest. One aspect that usually undergoes significant change is our sexual life. However, it's essential to recognize that intimacy can remain vibrant and fulfilling well into the senior years. Rediscovering each other emotionally and physically can be a powerful tool in rekindling the flame of passion. In this section, we delve into the importance of rediscovering each other and how it can enhance your sexual life.

1. **Building Emotional Connection**: Emotional intimacy forms the foundation of a healthy sexual relationship. For a couple who has been in a marriage for decades, the emotional connection may have diminished significantly. The many years of shared experiences, challenges, and triumphs can sometimes lead to complacency. Rediscovering each other emotionally involves actively listening, expressing appreciation, and nurturing a deeper understanding of one another. Engaging in meaningful conversations, reminiscing about shared memories, reflecting on the love you felt for each other when you first met and started dating, deciding to experiment with sleeping in the same bed together again and exploring new interests

together can reignite the emotional flame that may seem to have burned out.

2. **Prioritizing Physical Touch**: We can never over-emphasize or say enough about the fact that physical touch plays a crucial role in maintaining intimacy, regardless of age. However, as a couple grows older, changes in health and body image may affect their comfort level with physical affection. Rediscovering each other through touch involves gentle gestures, such as a massage, a back rub, or rubbing your mate's feet can evoke feelings of warmth and security. Gentle foreplay, without the expectation of actual intercourse, can be very stimulating. Your mate should feel free to touch or be touched by you without having the anxiety that it will lead to your demanding intercourse. Couples can also participate in activities like dancing, which promote physical closeness and arousal.

3. **Open Communication**: Effective communication is key to addressing any concerns or insecurities that may arise regarding intimacy. Openly discussing desires, preferences, and boundaries fosters a safe and supportive environment where both partners feel valued and understood. Rediscovering each other through communication involves actively listening without judgment, being vulnerable, and expressing affection verbally. You can also benefit from seeking guidance from therapists or counselors specializing in sexual health for seniors, who can offer personalized strategies and advice.

4. **Exploring New Horizons:** Exploring new experiences together can reignite passion and excitement in a long-term relationship. For a couple who has been together for many years, rediscovering each other may involve stepping outside of their comfort zones and embracing novelty. This could include trying new activities, embarking on adventures, or even experimenting with different sexual techniques or fantasies. By maintaining a sense of curiosity and openness to new possibilities, you can inject freshness and spontaneity into your sex life, enhancing satisfaction and connection.

5. **Nurturing Self-Care**: As previously stated, self-care is an essential aspect of rediscovering each other and improving sexual health.

Prioritizing physical well-being through regular exercise, nutritious eating habits, and adequate rest can boost energy levels and overall vitality. We should not overlook the importance of regularly taking a shower or bathing and good dental hygiene. It is hard to be sexually interested in a person with a body odor or bad breath. As men, we are usually the culprits in these matters. Also, you should wear appealing appropriate clean clothes, especially when out together in public. Wearing a sensual cologne or perfume can also stimulate your mate's sexual desire.

For a senior couple who has been together for years, over time, it's easy to fall into routines and forget the excitement of discovering each other. Rediscovering your partner can reignite passion and intimacy. Here are three things you can do to rediscover your partner:

1. **Date Nights**: Plan regular date nights to break the routine and create special memories. It doesn't have to be elaborate – a quiet dinner or a movie night can be just as meaningful.
2. **Travel Together**: Exploring new places and experiences can bring a sense of adventure and novelty to your relationship.
3. **Learn Together**: Take up a new hobby or class together. Learning something new can be a bonding experience and give you fresh topics to discuss and enjoy.

By focusing on these aspects of intimacy, you can create a deeper, more fulfilling relationship that enhances both your emotional and sexual connection. Remember, intimacy is a journey, not a destination, and every step you take towards understanding and loving each other more deeply enriches your shared life.

Conclusion:
Rediscovering each other emotionally and physically is a journey of exploration, growth, and reconnection. By nurturing emotional intimacy, prioritizing physical touch, fostering open communication, exploring new experiences, and practicing self-care, the two of you can revitalize your sexual life and strengthen your bond. Embracing this journey with curiosity, compassion, and a willingness to grow together can lead to a more fulfilling and satisfying relationship for you and your mate.

Chapter 6: Practical Tips and Techniques

In the first five chapters of this guide, we have discussed ways to improve your sexual life as a senior citizen. We have pointed out that the key to a happy sex life in your senior years involves understanding the changes that occur with age and finding practical strategies to adapt and enhance intimacy. Here is a summary of some practical tips and techniques we have discussed thus far:

1. **Communication:** Open and honest communication is key. Discuss desires, concerns, and any physical limitations without judgment. This fosters trust and understanding, paving the way for a satisfying sexual relationship.

2. **Health and Fitness:** Prioritize overall health and fitness. Regular exercise improves stamina, flexibility, and mood, all of which contribute to a better sex life. Consult a healthcare provider for personalized advice on exercise and nutrition.

3. **Medical Considerations:** Address any medical issues or medications that may affect sexual function. Many health conditions common in seniors, such as diabetes or cardiovascular disease, can impact sexual health. Seek medical advice for managing these conditions effectively.

4. **Exploration and Experimentation:** Embrace creativity and explore new ways to experience pleasure together. Experiment with different positions, techniques, and sensations. Keep an open mind and be willing to try new things.

5. **Sensate Focus:** Sensate focus exercises involve non-genital touch and can help you and your mate reconnect and build intimacy. Take time to explore each other's bodies without the pressure of sexual performance.

6. **Relaxation Techniques:** Stress and anxiety can interfere with sexual function. Practice relaxation techniques such as deep

breathing, meditation, or yoga to reduce tension and promote a more relaxed state of mind.

7. **Sensory Stimulation:** Engage all the senses to enhance arousal and pleasure. Utilize mood lighting, scented candles, soft music, and luxurious fabrics to create a sensual atmosphere.

8. **Foreplay:** Invest time in foreplay to increase arousal and build anticipation. Focus on kissing, caressing, and other forms of sensual touch to enhance intimacy and pleasure.

9. **Adaptation:** Be flexible and willing to adapt to changes in sexual function or desire. Explore alternative forms of intimacy, such as cuddling, kissing, or mutual massage, to maintain connection and closeness.

10. **Professional Help:** If difficulties persist, consider seeking help from a qualified sex therapist or counselor specializing in issues related to aging and sexuality. They can provide guidance, support, and practical techniques tailored to your specific needs.

By implementing these practical tips and techniques, you and your partner can cultivate a happy, fulfilling, and satisfying sex life.

Positioning and Comfort

We have already spoken about the fact that as we age, our bodies undergo various changes, including those that affect our sexual health and intimacy. We have learned from previous discussions in this guide that as seniors, maintaining a satisfying and fulfilling sexual life can become more challenging due to factors such as physical limitations, and medical conditions. Aging also brings about a range of additional physical changes that can impact sexual activity. Conditions such as arthritis, osteoporosis, and mobility issues may affect flexibility and comfort during sexual intercourse. Also, we have learned that hormonal changes, including decreased estrogen and testosterone levels, can lead to changes in libido and sexual function. However, despite the challenges, by focusing on positioning and comfort, we as seniors can continue to enjoy sex.

Importance of Positioning: Choosing the right sexual positions can significantly enhance comfort and pleasure for a senior citizen couple. Opting for positions that minimize strain on joints and muscles can alleviate discomfort and allow for more enjoyable intimacy. For example, positions that require less physical exertion, such as side-by-side or spooning positions, can be more comfortable for individuals with mobility issues or chronic pain.

Furthermore, experimenting with different positions allows a couple to find what works best for them and their unique physical abilities. Open communication and a willingness to explore new techniques can help you and your mate maintain a fulfilling sex life despite age-related physical challenges.

Prioritizing Comfort: Comfort is paramount when it comes to sexual intimacy in our senior years. This involves creating a conducive environment that promotes relaxation and reduces anxiety or discomfort. Simple adjustments, such as using extra pillows for support or ensuring adequate lubrication, can significantly enhance comfort during sexual activity.

Moreover, addressing any underlying medical conditions or concerns is crucial for optimizing comfort and safety. Consulting with healthcare professionals, such as physicians or physical therapists, can provide valuable guidance on managing health issues that may impact sexual function.

Communication and Connection: Again, communication is the key. In addition to focusing on positioning and comfort, effective communication is necessary to maintain intimacy in a senior-citizen relationship. Openly discussing desires, concerns, and preferences fosters trust and understanding, and will allow you and your mate to navigate any challenges together.

Conclusion:
While aging may present certain challenges to sexual intimacy, it by no means diminishes the potential for a fulfilling and satisfying sexual relationship. By prioritizing positioning and comfort, along with open communication and emotional connection, you can continue to enjoy sex. With patience, understanding, and a willingness to explore, you and your partner can continue to have a happy, healthy sex life for years to come.

Lubrication and Aids

As a senior citizen couple, maintaining a satisfying and fulfilling sex life may require some adjustments and adaptations. Among these, the use of lubrication and aids can play a crucial role in enhancing intimacy and pleasure. While some may feel hesitant or embarrassed to discuss these topics, it's important to recognize the significant benefits they can offer in improving sexual experiences for older adults.

As all of us as senior citizens know, aging brings about various physiological changes. And as we have previously discussed, these changes can impact our sexual health. We have learned in prior chapters of this guide, that both men and women may experience a decrease in hormone levels, changes in genital sensitivity, and conditions such as arthritis or diabetes that can affect mobility and overall comfort during sexual activity. These changes can lead to challenges such as vaginal dryness, erectile dysfunction, or difficulty achieving arousal and orgasm.

The Role of Lubrication: Lubrication is essential for comfortable and pleasurable sexual activity at any age, but it becomes especially important as we get older. Vaginal dryness, a common issue among menopausal and post-menopausal women, can cause discomfort, irritation, and pain during intercourse. Using a high-quality lubricant can alleviate these symptoms, making sex more enjoyable and reducing the risk of injury or tearing.

For older men experiencing erectile difficulties, lubricants can also be beneficial during manual stimulation or when using sex toys or aids. They can reduce friction and enhance sensations, helping to maintain arousal and achieve orgasm.

Aids and Enhancements: In addition to lubrication, you may also benefit from using various aids and enhancements to overcome physical limitations and to increase sexual pleasure. For example, using ergonomic pillows or cushions can provide better support and comfort during sex, particularly for individuals with joint pain or mobility issues. Vibrators or other sex toys can also add excitement and stimulation, making up for decreased sensitivity or erectile function.

Overcoming Stigma and Taboos: Despite the clear benefits, many seniors may feel hesitant to discuss lubrication, sex toys, and other aids due to stigma or embarrassment surrounding aging and sexuality. It's essential to break down these barriers and promote open, honest conversations about sexual health and intimacy among older adults. You should feel comfortable discussing and exploring these aids together with your mate. By doing so, you may discover new ways to experience pleasure and intimacy such as you have never experienced before. Healthcare providers can also play a crucial role in this process by providing education, resources, and support tailored to your comfort level.

Conclusion:

Maintaining a satisfying and fulfilling sex life is possible at any age, but it may require some adjustments and adaptations as we grow older. Lubrication, sex toys, and aids can be invaluable tools for enhancing intimacy, pleasure, and comfort. By embracing these tools and overcoming stigma, you can continue to enjoy fulfilling and meaningful sexual experiences throughout your life.

Addressing Erectile Dysfunction and Vaginal Dryness

With the numerous changes, our bodies go through as we age, maintaining a satisfying and fulfilling sex life becomes increasingly challenging due to conditions such as erectile dysfunction (ED) and vaginal dryness. However, addressing these issues is crucial for promoting overall well-being, intimacy, and emotional connection.

Erectile dysfunction, characterized by the inability to achieve or sustain an erection firm enough for sexual intercourse, is a common concern among aging men. It can be caused by various factors, including reduced blood flow to the penis, hormonal changes, medication side effects, and underlying health conditions such as diabetes or heart disease. Similarly, vaginal dryness, a condition in which the vaginal walls lack proper lubrication, is prevalent among menopausal and postmenopausal women due to hormonal fluctuations. The impact of these conditions on the sexual lives of those of us in our senior years can be profound. Feelings of frustration, embarrassment, and inadequacy may arise, leading us to a decline in sexual desire and intimacy. Moreover, unresolved sexual issues can strain a relationship and contribute to emotional distance between us and our partner. Some couples have actually divorced because their partner was no longer interested in sex.

Recognizing the importance of addressing ED and vaginal dryness is the first step toward improving your sexual wellness. By seeking medical guidance and exploring available treatment options, you can regain confidence and reignite passion in your relationship.

For men experiencing erectile dysfunction, treatments using oral medications such as Viagra, Cialis, Levitra, or Blue Chew. Also, penis injections, a vacuum device, or surgery may be recommended, depending on the underlying cause and individual health status.

Similarly, women dealing with vaginal dryness can benefit from various interventions aimed at restoring moisture and elasticity to the vaginal tissues. Over-the-counter lubricants and moisturizers can provide temporary relief, while hormone therapy or vaginal estrogen treatments may offer longer-term solutions by addressing underlying hormonal imbalances.

In addition to medical interventions, communication and mutual support between you and your partner are essential components of addressing sexual issues. Open and honest discussions about concerns, preferences, and desires can help alleviate anxiety and foster a deeper emotional connection.

Furthermore, as previously discussed in this guide, embracing a holistic approach to sexual wellness that prioritizes overall health and well-being can have far-reaching benefits. This includes maintaining a healthy lifestyle, staying physically active, managing stress effectively, and nurturing emotional intimacy outside the bedroom.

By acknowledging and addressing issues such as erectile dysfunction and vaginal dryness, as a couple, you can reclaim your sexual vitality and enjoy a fulfilling and intimate relationship. With the right support, guidance, and mindset, your love and passion for each other can thrive at any stage of life—regardless of how long it has been since the two of you have had sex together.

Chapter 7: Adapting to Physical Limitations

As society continues to evolve, so does our understanding of sexuality and intimacy across all age groups. And as we continue to promote open and inclusive discussions about senior sexuality, we pave the way for a more accepting and supportive society for all. Sexuality is a fundamental aspect of human nature, transcending age boundaries. However, as we age, we may encounter physical limitations that can pose challenges to maintaining a satisfying sexual relationship. As a senior citizen, adapting to these limitations becomes crucial in nurturing intimacy and preserving a happy sex life.

By embracing creativity, communication, and openness, you can navigate the challenges and explore new avenues of intimacy. By embracing adaptation, you and your mate can discover new ways to experience pleasure and intimacy and foster a deeper connection with each other. Through adaptation and innovation, age should never be a barrier to experiencing pleasure and connection in the realm of sexuality. In this chapter, we explore the importance of adaptation in overcoming barriers that may affect your sexual relationship.

Sexual Aids and Devices

Adapting to physical limitations often involves exploring alternative forms of intimacy beyond traditional sexual intercourse. We have already spoken about the importance of sensual massage, cuddling, kissing, and mutual masturbation, which provide opportunities for emotional connection and pleasure without placing undue strain on the body. However, in addition to these traditional alternatives, innovative assistive devices and aids can also play a valuable role in overcoming physical limitations and enhancing sexual pleasure. Devices such as ergonomic pillows, vibrators, lubricants, and erection aids can help address common challenges such as limited mobility and erectile dysfunction. By incorporating these tools into your sexual repertoire, you and your mate can reclaim joy and spontaneity in your intimate lives.

For a couple facing persistent challenges related to physical limitations, seeking professional guidance from healthcare providers or sex therapists can be immensely beneficial. These professionals can offer specialized advice, exercises, and treatments tailored to address your specific concerns and improve your sexual functioning. With the right support, you and your mate can overcome obstacles and rediscover the joy of intimacy.

Sexual Aids:
Sexual aids refer to products or devices that assist couples in enhancing their sexual experiences or overcoming specific challenges. These aids can range from therapeutic items to accessories that facilitate various sexual activities. Some examples:

1. **Erectile Dysfunction Aids**: Devices like vacuum erection devices (VEDs) or penile implants are used to achieve or maintain an erection.

2. **Lubricants**: Products used to reduce friction during sexual activity, enhancing comfort and pleasure. They come in water-based, silicone-based, and oil-based formulations.

3. **Sexual Enhancers**: Supplements or medications (prescribed or over-the-counter) aimed at boosting libido, increasing arousal, or improving sexual performance.

4. **Contraceptives**: Products like condoms, diaphragms, or intrauterine devices (IUDs) used to prevent pregnancy or sexually transmitted infections (STIs).

5. **Fertility Aids**: Devices or supplements designed to aid conception, such as fertility monitors or lubricants formulated to support sperm viability.

6. **Sexual Wellness Products**: Includes items like vaginal dilators (used to gradually stretch the vaginal walls), pelvic floor exercisers (to strengthen pelvic muscles), or Kegel balls (used for pelvic floor exercises and pleasure).

7. **Sexual Education Tools**: Books, videos, or online resources aimed at providing information and guidance on sexual health, techniques, and relationships.

8. **Sexual Hygiene Products**: Items like intimate washes, wipes, or odor-control products are designed to maintain cleanliness and freshness during sexual activities.

9. **Sexual Positioning Aids**: Cushions, ramps, or wedges designed to support and enhance comfort during different sexual positions.

10. **Sexual Health Screening Kits**: Home testing kits for STIs or fertility testing, allow individuals to monitor their sexual health privately.

These aids are intended to support sexual health, pleasure, and intimacy, and their use should be based on individual needs and preferences. It's important to consult healthcare professionals for guidance on choosing and using sexual aids safely and effectively.

Sex Devices:

Sex devices, also known as sex toys or adult toys, encompass a wide range of products designed to enhance sexual pleasure and exploration. Here are some common types of sex devices:

1. **Vibrators**: Electric or battery-powered devices that produce vibrations to stimulate erogenous zones such as the clitoris, vagina, or penis. They come in various shapes, sizes, and strengths, including bullet vibrators, wand vibrators, and rabbit vibrators.

2. **Dildos**: Phallic-shaped objects used for penetration. Dildos can be made from silicone, rubber, glass, or other materials. They vary in size, shape, and texture to cater to different preferences.

3. **Anal Toys**: Devices specifically designed for anal stimulation. This category includes butt plugs (small plugs inserted into the anus), anal beads (graduated beads for insertion and removal), and anal vibrators or prostate massagers (devices targeting the prostate gland).

4. **Male Masturbators**: Devices designed for solo male pleasure, often featuring textured sleeves or vibrating elements to simulate the sensations of vaginal, oral, or anal sex.

5. **Female Masturbators**: Devices designed for solo female pleasure, such as clitoral stimulators, G-spot vibrators, or suction toys that mimic oral sex sensations.

6. **Cock Rings**: Rings worn around the base of the penis (and sometimes the testicles) to enhance erection, stamina, and sensitivity by restricting blood flow.

7. **Kegel Balls**: Also known as Ben Wa balls or pleasure balls, these are used for pelvic floor exercises to strengthen the muscles and potentially enhance sexual pleasure.

8. **Remote-Controlled Toys**: Vibrators, dildos, or other devices that can be controlled remotely via a wireless connection or smartphone app, allowing partners to interact from a distance.

9. **Bondage Gear**: Equipment used in BDSM (Bondage, Discipline, Dominance, Submission, Sadism, Masochism) play, including restraints (such as handcuffs, ropes, or bondage tape), blindfolds, gags, and spanking implements.

10. **Sex Furniture**: Specialized furniture designed to facilitate various sexual positions and activities, such as sex swings, erotic chairs, or inclined beds.

11. **Sensation Play Devices**: Items designed to enhance sensory experiences during sex, such as feather ticklers, ice cubes, or wax play candles.

Conclusion:
These devices are meant to be used consensually to explore and enhance sexual experiences. And only with the consent of both parties should a sex device be used during any sexual activity. Nothing should ever be done that makes your partner feel ashamed or degraded. It is also essential that you and

your mate prioritize safety, cleanliness, and communication when incorporating sex devices into your sexual activities.

Sexual Function and Pleasure

Aging often brings physical challenges that can impact sexual function and pleasure. This is where sexual aids and devices play a crucial role. Sexual aids and devices, often stigmatized and misunderstood, can play an important role in supporting and revitalizing your intimacy. They can not only enhance physical pleasure but also reinforce trust, knowing that your partner will not do anything to harm or belittle you. Sexual aids and devices can also improve emotional connections, and foster a deeper bond between you and your mate. For a senior couple struggling to regain sexual intimacy, sexual aids and devices could be beneficial physically, emotionally, psychologically, and socially.

Physical Benefits:

1. **Addressing Erectile Dysfunction** - Erectile dysfunction (ED) is a common issue among older men. Devices such as cock rings, vacuum erection devices (VEDs), and penile implants can significantly improve erectile function, allowing for sustained intimacy. These aids provide a non-pharmaceutical solution that can be used as needed, giving a couple the spontaneity and confidence to engage in sexual activities.

2. **Alleviating Vaginal Dryness** - Post-menopausal women often experience vaginal dryness, which can make intercourse uncomfortable or painful. Lubricants and vaginal moisturizers are simple yet effective solutions that can enhance comfort and pleasure during sexual activity. Additionally, vaginal dilators can help maintain vaginal elasticity and health.

3. **Supporting Mobility Issues** - For a couple with mobility limitations, positioning aids such as wedges or supportive cushions can facilitate more comfortable and varied sexual positions. These aids can reduce physical strain and make sex more accessible and enjoyable.

Emotional Benefits:

1. **Enhancing Intimacy** - Sexual aids and devices such as vibrators and stimulators can enhance sexual pleasure for both partners. Sexual toys can reignite the spark in a relationship by introducing new sensations and experiences. Exploring these toys together encourages communication, trust, and mutual understanding. This shared exploration fosters a deeper emotional connection, promoting a sense of closeness and bonding that transcends physical pleasure. These devices can be particularly beneficial in countering the decreased sensitivity that often accompanies aging. They provide varied and intense sensations that can lead to more satisfying sexual experiences.

2. **Boosting Confidence and Self-Esteem** - Using sexual aids and devices can help you feel more confident in your ability to engage in sexual activity. This boost in confidence can translate to a more positive self-image and a stronger desire for intimacy.

3. **Strengthening Relationship** - The shared experience of exploring sexual aids and devices can enhance communication and intimacy between you and your mate. Discussing preferences, trying new aids and devices, and discovering mutual pleasures can deepen emotional bonds and foster a sense of partnership.

4. **Promoting Open Communication** - Introducing sexual aids and devices into a relationship often necessitates open and honest communication. This dialogue can lead to a better understanding of each other's needs and desires, creating a more fulfilling sexual relationship.

Psychological Benefits:

1. **Reducing Anxiety and Stress** - Concerns about sexual performance can create anxiety and stress. For instance, the man may be worried about is he going to be able to get an erection. The woman may be worried about whether the penetration is going to be painful. Sexual aids and devices offer practical solutions that can alleviate

these worries, allowing you and your partner to focus on enjoying your time together rather than on potential difficulties.

2. **Boosting Confidence** - The use of sexual aids and devices can boost confidence and self-esteem among senior citizens. As we experience enhanced sexual pleasure and satisfaction, our overall sense of well-being improves. This newfound confidence often extends beyond the bedroom, positively impacting other areas of our lives.

Social Benefits:

1. **Breaking Taboos** - Discussing and using aids and devices can help break down societal taboos surrounding senior sexuality. By openly embracing your sexual desires and needs, as an older adult, you will be challenging your own and society's stereotypes about older adults and sexuality. Embracing your sexual self will also give you a more inclusive understanding of your sexual needs and desires. This shift in perspective benefits not only you and your mate but also society as a whole, promoting a culture of acceptance and respect for diverse sexual experiences.

2. **Embracing Change** - Despite the clear benefits, there remains a stigma surrounding the use of sexual aids, particularly among older adults. It is essential to challenge these taboos and recognize that sexual health is a vital aspect of overall well-being at any age. Healthcare professionals and support groups can play a pivotal role in educating and normalizing the use of sexual aids, thus encouraging you to embrace these tools as part of your sexual wellness.

A Practical Consideration:

Safety and Comfort - When selecting sexual aids and devices, it is crucial to prioritize safety and comfort. Access to accurate information and resources is essential when exploring sexual toys. You should opt for high-quality, body-safe materials and designs that cater to your specific needs. Consulting with healthcare professionals or sex therapists can provide valuable guidance in choosing appropriate products.

Conclusion:

Sexual aids and devices are invaluable tools that can significantly enhance your sexual relationship. By addressing physical challenges and enhancing pleasure, these aids and devices contribute to a more satisfying and fulfilling intimate life. Moreover, the emotional benefits, such as increased confidence and strengthened relationships, underscore their importance. Embracing sexual aids and devices can lead to a richer, more connected, and joyful experience, and support in both physical and emotional well-being. Sexual aids and devices also hold significant potential in enhancing the sexual relationships of you and your mate. By addressing physical changes, enhancing intimacy, boosting confidence, and challenging societal taboos, these items can contribute to you and your mate having a fulfilling and vibrant sex life.

Alternative Sexual Practices

Alternative sexual practices play a crucial role in improving the sexual relationships of senior citizen couples. By embracing change, communicating openly, and exploring diverse forms of intimacy, as an older adult, you can maintain a vibrant and satisfying sexual connection. These practices not only enhance physical pleasure but also strengthen emotional bonds, contributing to a happier and healthier life in your senior years—in and out of the bedroom.

As has already been stated on several occasions throughout this guide, as we age, our bodies undergo various changes that can affect our sexual relationships. Aging can bring about physical challenges such as decreased libido, erectile dysfunction, vaginal dryness, and reduced stamina. These changes, however, do not signify the end of a fulfilling sex life. Instead, they present an opportunity to explore new and alternative sexual practices that can revitalize intimacy. These changes often require adjustments and adaptations to maintain a fulfilling and intimate connection. Alternative sexual practices offer a pathway to sustaining and even enhancing our sexual relationship, fostering intimacy, emotional connection, trust, and overall well-being.

Embracing your body's changes with openness and creativity can lead to deeper emotional bonds and a renewed sense of closeness with your partner. However, effective communication is the cornerstone of any successful sexual relationship, especially for a senior couple exploring alternative practices. Discussing desires, preferences, and boundaries openly can help you and your mate understand each other better and create a safe space for experimentation. This dialogue can also alleviate anxieties or misconceptions about aging and sexuality, allowing the two of you to focus on your shared experiences and mutual satisfaction. Below is a list of three alternative practices you may wish to explore.

Exploring Alternative Practices:

1. Sensate Focus Exercises: Sensate focus exercises, a cornerstone of sex therapy, involve non-genital touch and caressing, focusing on sensation rather than performance. These exercises can help you and your partner reconnect physically and emotionally without the pressure of traditional sexual intercourse.

2. Tantric and Mindfulness: Tantric practices and mindfulness in sex emphasize prolonged and meaningful physical connection. By focusing on breathing, eye contact, and synchronized movements, as a couple, you can create a deeply intimate and spiritual experience.

3. Role-Playing and Fantasies: Exploring fantasies and engaging in role-playing can add excitement and novelty to the relationship. It allows you and your mate to break away from routine and rediscover each other in new and exhilarating ways.

Conclusion:
Alternative sexual practices play a critical role in improving the sexual relationships of a senior citizen couple. By embracing change, communicating openly, and exploring diverse forms of intimacy, you and your mate can maintain a vibrant and satisfying sexual connection. These

practices not only enhance physical pleasure but also strengthen emotional bonds, contributing to a happier sex life in your senior years.

Mindfulness and Sensuality

Aging often brings a host of physical and emotional changes that can impact intimacy and sexual relationships. For a senior citizen couple, maintaining a happy fulfilling sexual connection can be challenging yet profoundly rewarding. Mindfulness and sensuality play crucial roles in enhancing intimacy and revitalizing the sexual experiences of older adults. By fostering presence, emotional connection, and a deeper appreciation for physical sensations, mindfulness, and sensuality can significantly improve the sexual relationship between you and your partner.

Understanding Mindfulness:
Mindfulness is the practice of being fully present in the moment, and aware of one's thoughts, feelings, and bodily sensations without judgment. It encourages you and your mate to focus on the here and now, fostering a deeper connection with yourself and your partner. In the context of a sexual relationship, mindfulness can help you become more attuned to your needs and desires, creating a more intimate and satisfying sexual experience.

The Role of Sensuality:
Sensuality involves the appreciation and enjoyment of the body's sensory experiences. Unlike sexuality, which focuses on sexual activity and desire, sensuality emphasizes touch, taste, smell, sight, and sound to enhance intimacy. For a senior couple, exploring sensuality can lead to a richer and more varied sexual relationship. It shifts the focus from performance and specific outcomes to the enjoyment of shared experiences and connections.

The Intersection of Mindfulness and Sensuality:
When mindfulness and sensuality are combined, they create a powerful synergy that can transform your sexual relationship. Here are some key benefits:

1. Enhanced Emotional Connection
Mindfulness fosters emotional presence and empathy, allowing partners to connect on a deeper level. By being fully present during intimate moments,

as a couple, you can communicate more effectively and understand each other's emotional and physical needs better. This deeper emotional connection can enhance trust and intimacy, creating a more fulfilling sexual relationship.

2. Reduced Anxiety and Stress
Performance anxiety and stress can negatively impact sexual experiences. Mindfulness helps reduce these feelings by encouraging each of you to focus on the present moment rather than worrying about past experiences or future expectations. This relaxed state of mind can lead to more enjoyable and spontaneous sexual encounters.

3. Heightened Sensory Awareness
Sensuality involves engaging all the senses to enhance intimacy. When combined with mindfulness, this heightened sensory awareness allows you and your mate to fully immerse yourselves in the sensory experiences of touch, taste, smell, sound, and sight. This can make sexual activities more pleasurable and meaningful.

4. Improved Physical Comfort
Aging can bring physical changes that affect sexual comfort and pleasure. Mindfulness encourages a gentle and accepting approach to these changes. You and your mate can explore new ways of experiencing pleasure that are comfortable for both partners. Sensual activities, such as massage or simply holding hands, can be deeply satisfying and intimate.

5. Rekindling Passion
Routine and familiarity can sometimes dampen sexual passion. Mindfulness and sensuality encourage exploration and novelty within the relationship. By focusing on the present moment and appreciating each other's bodies and sensations, you can rekindle the passion and excitement that may have waned over the years.

Practical Tips for A Senior Couple

Incorporating mindfulness and sensuality into a sexual relationship requires practice and openness. Here is a review of some practical mindfulness and sensuality tips, several of which we have previously discussed in this guide:

1. Practice Mindful Breathing

Before engaging in sexual activities, take a few minutes to practice mindful breathing together. This helps in calming the mind and creating a sense of presence and connection.

2. Engage in Sensory Exploration

Spend time exploring each other's bodies through touch, focusing on the sensations rather than specific goals. Use different textures, temperatures, and types of touch to enhance the sensory experience.

3. Communicate Openly

Discuss your desires, fears, and preferences openly and without judgment. Communication is key to understanding each other's needs and enhancing intimacy.

4. Create a Relaxing Environment

Set the mood by creating a relaxing environment. Soft lighting, soothing music, and scented candles can enhance the sensory experience and create a comfortable space for intimacy.

5. Take Your Time

There's no rush. Take your time to enjoy each other's company and the shared experience. Focus on the journey rather than the destination.

Conclusion:

Mindfulness and sensuality offer powerful tools to enhance your sexual relationship. By fostering presence, deepening emotional connections, and appreciating the richness of sensory experiences, these practices can help us as older adults to navigate the changes that come with aging and maintain a fulfilling and intimate sexual connection. Embracing mindfulness and sensuality can lead to a more satisfying and enriching relationship, proving that passion, intimacy, and a happy sex life can thrive at any age.

Chapter 8: Staying Safe

Staying safe in a sexual relationship is a multifaceted approach involving physical health, emotional well-being, and mutual respect. By prioritizing safety, you can continue to enjoy a happy sex life. Open communication, regular health checkups, exercising, eating healthy, and a willingness to explore and adapt can make the golden years truly golden in every sense.

As we age, maintaining a fulfilling and safe sexual relationship becomes an essential aspect of overall well-being and quality of life. For a senior citizen couple, the importance of staying safe while engaging in sexual activities cannot be overstated. Ensuring safety in this intimate aspect of life not only protects physical health but also fosters emotional connection, trust, and mutual respect. Here are four areas of concern where staying safe is crucial for a happy sex life:

1. Physical Health and Safety:

    a. **Managing Health Conditions** - Many of us seniors live with chronic conditions such as heart disease, diabetes, or arthritis. These conditions can affect sexual performance and enjoyment. Consulting healthcare providers to manage these conditions and discussing any potential impact on sexual activity is vital.

    b. **Medication Interactions** - Certain medications can affect sexual function. Understanding how prescribed drugs interact with sexual health is essential. Healthcare providers can adjust medications or suggest alternatives to minimize negative impacts on sexual activity.

2. Emotional and Psychological Well-being:

    a. **Communication** - Open and honest communication about desires, boundaries, and health concerns is central. Discussing these topics fosters trust and ensures both partners feel comfortable and respected.

b. **Consent and Comfort** - Ensuring that both partners are comfortable and consensual in all sexual activities is fundamental. Respecting each other's limits and preferences leads to a more satisfying and safe sexual experience.

c. **Addressing Psychological Barriers** - Aging can bring about body image concerns or anxiety related to sexual performance. Seeking counseling or therapy can help address these issues, enabling you and your mate to enjoy a healthier and more confident sexual relationship.

3. Enhancing Intimacy and Connection:

a. **Quality Over Quantity** - As physical abilities change with age, focusing on the quality of intimate moments rather than frequency can enhance satisfaction. Exploring different ways to express love and intimacy, such as holding hands, snuggling, going on walks, or simply spending quality time together, can be deeply fulfilling.

b. **Experimenting Safely** - Trying new things can keep the sexual relationship exciting. However, it's important to ensure that any new activities are safe. For instance, using appropriate lubricants can prevent discomfort or injury, and ensuring a safe and comfortable environment can enhance the experience.

c. **Education and Resources** - Accessing educational resources about sexual health in later life can empower couples. Many organizations provide valuable information tailored to senior sexual health, helping couples navigate changes and maintain a healthy sexual relationship.

4. The Role of Support Systems:

a. **Healthcare Providers** - Regular check-ups with a healthcare provider specializing in geriatric care can provide tailored advice and address any sexual health concerns.

b. **Support Groups** - Joining support groups for seniors can offer a platform to share experiences and learn from others facing similar challenges. This can also reduce feelings of isolation and enhance emotional well-being.

c. **Community Resources** - Many communities offer resources and workshops on senior sexual health. Participating in these can provide valuable insights to strengthen your relationship with your mate.

Safe Sex Practices

As we age, our sexual health continues to play a vital role in our overall well-being and quality of life. For a senior citizen couple, maintaining an active and satisfying sexual relationship can enhance intimacy, emotional connection, and physical health. However, it is crucial to prioritize safe sex practices to ensure that these benefits are enjoyed without compromising health. Below are some important safe sex practices and how you and your mate can improve your sexual relationship.

1. **Understanding the Need for Safe Sex Practices**
   Safe sex practices are often associated with younger populations, but they are equally important for senior citizens. The primary concerns include the prevention of Sexually Transmitted Infections (STIs), maintaining physical health, and ensuring emotional well-being.

2. **Physical Health Considerations**
   As the body ages, changes such as vaginal dryness for women and erectile dysfunction for men can affect sexual activity. These changes can increase the risk of injury or discomfort during sex. Using lubricants, engaging in gentle and patient sexual activities, and seeking medical advice for any concerns can help ensure a pleasurable and safe sexual experience.

3. **Physical Changes and Safe Sex**
   Some seniors may feel embarrassed or reluctant to address the physical changes that come with aging. It's important to normalize these conversations and seek appropriate medical advice and

products, such as lubricants or medications, to enhance sexual health and safety.

4. **Enhancing Emotional and Intimate Connection**
   A healthy sexual relationship can significantly enhance the emotional bond between you and your partner. Safe sex practices contribute to a sense of security and trust, allowing your partner and you to focus on your intimacy without fear or anxiety.

5. **Building Trust and Communication**
   Open and honest communication about sexual desires, boundaries, and health status fosters a deeper emotional connection. Discussing safe sex practices, such as condom use and regular health check-ups, can strengthen trust and ensure that you both feel respected and cared for.

6. **Reducing Anxiety and Stress**
   Health concerns can create stress and anxiety that interfere with sexual enjoyment. By prioritizing safe sex practices, you can alleviate these worries, leading to a more relaxed and fulfilling sexual relationship.

7. **Addressing Common Misconceptions**
   Many seniors may believe that safe sex is only necessary for younger individuals or those who are not in a long-term relationship. Dispelling these misconceptions is crucial for your personal safety and well-being.

Practical Tips for Safe Sex in a Senior Relationship

Here are some practical steps you and your partner can take to ensure your sexual health and safety:
- **Use Protection**: Condoms are effective in preventing most STIs. Female condoms or dental dams can also be used for additional protection.
- **Regular Health Checkups**: Both partners should undergo regular medical and STI screenings.

- **Communicate Openly**: Discuss sexual health openly and honestly with your partner and healthcare provider.
- **Stay Informed**: Educate yourself about the risks and prevention methods for STIs.
- **Consider Lubrication**: Use water-based lubricants to reduce discomfort and prevent injury during intercourse.

Conclusion:

Safe sex practices are a fundamental aspect of maintaining a healthy and satisfying sexual relationship with your partner. By prioritizing protection, open communication, and regular health checks, you and your mate can enjoy the emotional and physical benefits of a vibrant sexual connection. Embracing these practices not only enhances intimacy but also ensures that the joys of sexual activity are experienced safely and confidently.

Understanding and Preventing STIs

Contrary to common belief, sexually transmitted infections (STIs) are not exclusive to younger populations. The risk of STIs remains significant for sexually active seniors, especially those with a new or multiple partners. Using protection, such as a condom, and undergoing regular health screenings can prevent the spread of infections. You should make getting checked for STIs a regular part of your annual physical—especially if you have multiple partners.

As we age, the pursuit of a fulfilling and happy life remains a priority, and this includes maintaining a healthy and satisfying sexual relationship. As senior citizens, understanding and preventing sexually transmitted infections (STIs) is crucial not only for our physical health but also for enhancing our emotional and relational well-being. In this section, we will explore why understanding STIs is important for senior citizens and how prevention can lead to a happier and healthier sex life.

Preventing Sexually Transmitted Infections

STIs do not discriminate based on age. With the rise in dating and new relationships among seniors, the risk of STIs remains significant. According to the Centers for Disease Control and Prevention (CDC), rates of certain

STIs have been increasing among older adults. Safe sex practices, such as the use of condoms, regular STI screenings, and open communication about sexual health, are essential to prevent the spread of infections.

STIs and a Long-Term Relationship
Even in a long-term relationship, safe sex is important if one or both partners have had other sexual partners. Regular STI screenings and open discussions about sexual history are vital for maintaining health and safety.

The Prevalence of STIs Among Seniors
Contrary to common misconceptions, sexual activity remains a significant part of life for many senior citizens. Advances in healthcare, increased life expectancy, and the availability of treatments for erectile dysfunction and other sexual health issues mean that as seniors we can enjoy active sex lives well into our later years. However, this also means that we are not immune to the risks of STIs. In fact, the rates of STIs among us older adults have been rising. According to data from the Centers for Disease Control (CDC) and Prevention, the rates of syphilis, gonorrhea, and chlamydia have more than doubled among those of us 55 and older. Research also suggests that many of us older adults are unaware of these risks, and this is keeping us from adequate screening and practicing safer sex. This trend underscores the importance of education and prevention strategies tailored to our age group. Here are three reasons why as senior citizens we must be concerned about contracting STIs:

1. **Health Complications**: We are often more vulnerable to the health complications associated with STIs due to our age and possible pre-existing health conditions. Infections like HIV, syphilis, and gonorrhea can have severe effects on our health, leading to increased morbidity and mortality.

2. **Quality of Life**: The physical discomfort and emotional distress caused by STIs can significantly impact our quality of life. Pain, itching, odor, and other symptoms can interfere with daily activities and sleep, leading to a decrease in overall well-being.

3. **Relationship Dynamics**: The presence of an STI can strain a relationship. Feelings of guilt, shame, or blame can arise, causing emotional distance between you and your partner. Addressing and

preventing STIs can foster trust and intimacy, enhancing the emotional bond between you and your mate.

The Importance of Education and Communication

Education is the first line of defense against STIs. You should obtain accurate and comprehensive information about the risks, symptoms, and prevention methods of STIs. Healthcare providers play a crucial role in this regard by offering non-judgmental advice and resources. You can receive additional information and resources free of charge online at the U.S. Department of Health and Human Services (HHS) www.HHS.gov or your local health department.

Equally important is open communication between you and your partner. Communication! Communication! Communication! We can never emphasize this enough! Whether you are a man or a woman, discussing sexual health openly and honestly can strengthen your relationship and ensure that you and your mate are on the same page regarding prevention and treatment. This dialogue can also include discussing sexual histories, current health statuses, and the mutual decision to use protection such as condoms. Please be mindful that discussion about sex with your partner is not a one-and-done conversation—but it should be a regular part of your dialogue with one another. Below are some prevention strategies to help you and your mate reduce the possibility of contracting an STI.

Prevention Strategies for Senior Couples

1. **Regular Health Checkups**: Regular visits to healthcare providers for checkups and screenings are essential. Early detection of STIs can lead to more effective treatment and prevent the spread of infections.

2. **Safe Sex Practices**: Using condoms and other protective barriers can significantly reduce the risk of contracting STIs. Despite the fact that because of age, we generally no longer need a condom to prevent the risk of pregnancy—a condom is still useful for STI prevention.

3. **Vaccinations**: Vaccinations are available for certain STIs, such as the human papillomavirus (HPV). You should consult your

healthcare provider to determine which vaccines are appropriate for you.

4. **Healthy Lifestyle Choices**: Maintaining a healthy lifestyle through diet, exercise, and avoiding excessive alcohol or tobacco use can boost the immune system and overall health, making the body more resilient to infections.

Conclusion:

A healthy sex life contributes to overall happiness and well-being. As we celebrate our vitality and sexual health, let us also commit to empowering ourselves with the knowledge and tools we need in order to enjoy our golden years to the fullest. Understanding and preventing STIs is a critical component of the knowledge and tools we need for enjoying sex to the fullest and in maintaining a happy and healthy sex life in our golden years.

Through education, communication, and proactive health measures, you can protect yourself and your partner, leading to enhanced intimacy and emotional connection. Emotional intimacy and sexual satisfaction are interconnected, and both are vital for a strong relationship. By prioritizing sexual health and STI prevention, you and your mate can enjoy a more satisfying and intimate relationship, free from the anxiety and health risks associated with infections.

Regular Health Screenings

As we age, the intersection of physical health and sexual satisfaction becomes increasingly prominent. Regular health screenings play a crucial role in ensuring that both partners can continue to enjoy intimacy and a strong sexual relationship. Here are 7 reasons why regular health screenings are vital for a senior couple aiming to sustain a happy sex life.

1. Identifying and Managing Chronic Conditions

Chronic conditions such as diabetes, hypertension, and heart disease are common in us older adults and can significantly impact sexual function. For instance, diabetes can cause neuropathy and vascular issues, leading to erectile dysfunction in men and reduced lubrication and arousal in women.

Regular health screenings help in the early detection and management of these conditions, allowing for timely interventions that can mitigate their effects on sexual health.

2. Monitoring Hormonal Levels
Hormonal changes are a natural part of aging. In men, testosterone levels typically decline, which can lead to reduced libido and erectile issues. Women experience menopause, which brings about changes in estrogen and progesterone levels, potentially causing vaginal dryness, discomfort during intercourse, and a decrease in sexual desire. Through regular screenings, a healthcare provider can monitor these hormonal changes and suggest treatments such as hormone replacement therapy (HRT) or other medications that can help maintain a satisfying sex life.

3. Addressing Psychological Health
Mental health is intrinsically linked to sexual well-being. Conditions like depression, anxiety, and stress are known to affect sexual desire and performance. Regular health screenings often include evaluations of mental health, providing an opportunity to address any psychological barriers to a fulfilling sex life. Counseling, therapy, and medication can be effective treatments to enhance mental well-being and, consequently, sexual satisfaction.

4. Ensuring Medication Management
Many of us senior citizens take multiple medications, some of which can have side effects that interfere with sexual function. For example, certain blood pressure medications, antidepressants, and antipsychotics can lead to sexual dysfunction. Regular health screenings allow healthcare providers to review and adjust medications as needed, minimizing negative impacts on sexual health and ensuring that any medication-induced sexual issues are addressed promptly.

5. Promoting Healthy Lifestyle Choices
Health screenings often come with recommendations for lifestyle changes that can improve overall health and sexual function. As previously stated, regular exercise, a balanced diet, quitting smoking, and limiting alcohol intake are all factors that contribute to better sexual health. Maintaining a healthy lifestyle can enhance stamina, improve mood, and boost self-confidence, all of which are critical components of a satisfying sexual relationship.

6. Encouraging Open Communication

Health screenings can serve as a catalyst for open discussions between you, your partner, and your healthcare provider about sexual health. You might feel uncomfortable bringing up sexual issues, but regular checkups provide a structured environment to discuss these concerns. Open communication is key to identifying and addressing sexual health problems, ensuring both you and your partner feel heard and supported.

7. Preventing and Treating Sexual Health Conditions

Conditions such as erectile dysfunction, vaginal atrophy, and urinary incontinence can be common in us older adults and can severely impact sexual satisfaction. Regular screenings can help detect these issues early and provide treatments such as medications, pelvic floor exercises, or surgical options. Addressing these conditions promptly can prevent them from becoming barriers to a happy sex life.

Conclusion:

For a senior citizen couple, regular health screenings are not just about maintaining general health; they are pivotal in sustaining a happy and fulfilling sex life. By identifying and managing chronic conditions, monitoring hormonal levels, addressing psychological health, ensuring proper medication management, promoting healthy lifestyle choices, encouraging open communication, and preventing and treating sexual health conditions, regular health check-ups empower you and your mate to continue enjoying intimacy and connection. Investing in regular health screenings is an investment in a richer, more satisfying sexual relationship, contributing to your overall well-being and happiness.

Chapter 9: Mental and Emotional Well-Being

In the journey of life, the golden years are often viewed as a time for relaxation, reflection, and cherishing the accumulated experiences and memories. However, an aspect that sometimes goes overlooked in the lives of us senior citizens is the significance of maintaining a healthy and fulfilling sexual relationship. Contrary to common misconceptions, as stated previously in this guide, sexual intimacy is not just for the young; it remains a vital part of life for many of us as older adults. Central to achieving a happy sex life in our senior years is the cultivation of mental and emotional well-being.

The Interwovenness of a Happy Sex Life With Mental and Emotional Well-Being

The journey to a happy and fulfilling sex life in the senior years is deeply intertwined with mental and emotional well-being. By prioritizing emotional connection, addressing mental health concerns, and maintaining open communication, we can enjoy a rich and satisfying sexual relationship. The golden years offer a unique opportunity for us to explore new dimensions of intimacy for enhancing our overall happiness and quality of life, and opportunities to deepen our emotional bonds with our partner.

Mental and emotional well-being forms the cornerstone of a satisfying sexual relationship at any age, and it becomes even more critical in later years. Emotional connection and mental health significantly influence sexual desire, performance, and satisfaction. Understanding the link between mental and emotional health and sexual intimacy is important if you are truly seeking to have a happy sex life. Here's how these elements interplay to enhance your sexual relationship:

1. **Emotional Connection:**

   - **Strengthening Bonds** - Emotional intimacy deepens the bond between you and your mate, fostering a sense of security and trust. This trust is essential for open communication about desires, boundaries, and concerns, which enhances sexual satisfaction.

- **Reducing Anxiety** - Emotional closeness helps in alleviating anxieties related to sexual performance or changes in sexual function, which are common as we age. A supportive partner can provide reassurance, making sexual experiences more comfortable and enjoyable.

2. **Mental Health:**

- **Reducing Stress and Depression** - Mental health issues such as stress, anxiety, and depression can significantly impact libido and sexual satisfaction. Addressing these issues through therapy, mindfulness, or medication can lead to improved mental states and, consequently, a more fulfilling sex life.

- **Enhancing Self-Esteem** - Positive mental health contributes to higher self-esteem and body image. As a senior citizen, accepting and embracing the natural changes in your body can remove barriers to sexual enjoyment and intimacy.

Enhancing Mental and Emotional Well-Being

There are also several practical steps you can take to enhance your mental and emotional well-being. We have already discussed these steps in one form or another in other areas of this guide, such as open communication, living a healthy lifestyle, seeking professional help, mindfulness and relaxation techniques, and embracing change.

1. **Open Communication:**
- Engage in honest and open discussions about sexual needs, preferences, and any concerns. This transparency reduces misunderstandings and fosters a stronger emotional connection.

- Regularly share feelings and thoughts with each other, not just about sex but about life in general. This ongoing dialogue helps in maintaining a deep emotional bond.

2. **Healthy Lifestyle:**
   - Maintain a balanced diet, regular exercise, and adequate sleep. Physical health directly influences mental and emotional well-being, which in turn affects sexual health.
   - Engage in activities that bring joy and relaxation, whether it's hobbies, playing pickle ball, traveling, or spending time with the grandkids.

3. **Seeking Professional Help:**
   - Don't hesitate to seek therapy or counseling for mental health issues or sexual difficulties. Professionals can provide valuable guidance and support.
   - Sharing experiences and learning from others can be incredibly beneficial. Therefore, consider joining a support group or workshops that focus on sexual health and relationships for seniors.

4. **Mindfulness and Relaxation Techniques:**
   - Practices such as meditation, yoga, and deep-breathing exercises can reduce stress and enhance emotional well-being. These techniques help in creating a relaxed and open mindset conducive to intimacy.

5. **Embracing Changes:**
   - Accept and embrace the changes that come with aging. Understanding that sexual activity may evolve over time allows for a more adaptive and fulfilling sex life.
   - Explore different ways to express intimacy. Physical closeness, affectionate touch, reading a romance novel together, and non-sexual forms of intimacy can be equally satisfying and important.

Addressing Anxiety and Depression

We have learned throughout this guide that sexuality is a fundamental aspect of human life, and its significance doesn't diminish with age. As a senior citizen, maintaining a fulfilling sex life can contribute significantly to your overall happiness and relationship satisfaction. However, factors like anxiety and depression can often cast a shadow over intimacy, impacting both physical and emotional well-being. Addressing these mental health challenges is critical for promoting a vibrant and satisfying sexual relationship. Therefore, it is vital that you have an understanding of anxiety and depression as you continue to progress to a happy sex life throughout your senior years.

Understanding Anxiety and Depression in Seniors: Anxiety and depression are prevalent mental health issues among older adults, often overlooked or dismissed as a natural part of aging. However, these conditions can profoundly affect various aspects of our lives, including sexual intimacy. Anxiety may manifest as worry, fear, or nervousness, leading to performance anxiety or inhibitions in expressing desires. Depression, characterized by persistent sadness, loss of interest, and fatigue, can dampen libido and disrupt emotional connection.

Impact on Sexual Satisfaction: Anxiety and depression can significantly diminish your sexual satisfaction. Feelings of unease or apprehension can hinder arousal and enjoyment, while low mood and lack of energy may lead to disinterest in sexual activity altogether. Moreover, these mental health challenges can strain communication and intimacy, creating a cycle of frustration and dissatisfaction within your relationship.

Importance of Addressing Anxiety and Depression: Recognizing and addressing anxiety and depression are crucial steps in fostering a happy sex life. Seeking professional help, such as therapy or counseling, can provide valuable support in managing these mental health concerns. Therapeutic techniques, including cognitive-behavioral therapy (CBT) and mindfulness practices, can help you develop coping strategies, enhance self-esteem, and improve communication skills, thus revitalizing intimacy and sexual satisfaction. Also, your anxiety or depression may be due to a medical condition such as an improperly functioning thyroid. Your healthcare provider can run tests to determine the cause of your anxiety or depression and prescribe medication to help address your condition.

Enhancing Emotional Connection: Addressing anxiety and depression goes beyond alleviating symptoms; it involves nurturing emotional connection and intimacy within your relationship. Open and honest communication about your feelings, desires, and concerns creates a supportive environment where both you and your mate feel understood and valued. Building trust and intimacy through shared experiences, affectionate gestures, and mutual respect strengthens the emotional bond, laying the foundation for a fulfilling sexual relationship.

Exploring New Avenues of Intimacy: It can never be overemphasized the importance for you and your mate to explore alternative avenues of intimacy to enhance your sexual satisfaction. This may involve discovering new forms of physical affection, that prioritize emotional connection over performance. Experimenting with different activities, fantasies, or role-playing—such as dressing up as an ancient Egyptian queen or a superhero as a part of your sexual foreplay can reignite passion and creativity, fostering a sense of excitement and adventure in the bedroom.

Conclusion:
In the journey towards a happy sex life, addressing anxiety and depression is paramount. By acknowledging and managing these mental health challenges, you and your partner can cultivate emotional connections, enhance communication, and explore new avenues of intimacy, ultimately rekindling passion and satisfaction in your sexual relationship. With support, understanding, and a commitment to mutual well-being, the two of you can enjoy a lifelong vibrant, fulfilling, and happy sex life.

Boosting Self-Esteem and Body Image

Sexuality doesn't have an expiration date. However, aging does bring about various physical transformations, including changes in appearance, mobility, and sexual function. These changes can affect how we as seniors perceive ourselves and our bodies, leading to diminished self-esteem and body image concerns. Common issues such as weight gain, wrinkles, graying hair, loss of muscle tone, sagging breasts, a balding head, a potbelly, or a sexual dysfunction may contribute to feelings of inadequacy and self-consciousness, impacting sexual confidence and desire.

As seniors, maintaining a fulfilling sex life often requires us to navigate through these physical and emotional changes that come with aging. It is through fostering a positive sense of self and body image that play a significant role in revitalizing intimacy and enhancing our sexual satisfaction. In this section, we delve into the importance of self-esteem and body image in the context of a senior sexual relationship and explore strategies to boost self-esteem and body image for a more fulfilling intimate, and happier sex life.

The Interplay of Self-Esteem, Body Image, and Sexuality:

Self-esteem is defined as one's overall sense of self-worth and value. Your self-esteem heavily influences how you perceive your body and how you approach sexual intimacy. A healthy level of self-esteem fosters confidence, resilience, and a positive outlook on life, all of which are crucial for maintaining a satisfying sexual relationship. Conversely, low self-esteem can manifest as feelings of insecurity, anxiety, and reluctance to engage in sexual activity, thus hindering intimacy and enjoyment.

Body image is the subjective perception of one's physical appearance. It also plays a significant role in sexual well-being. A senior citizen who feels dissatisfied with his or her body may struggle to feel desirable or attractive, such as being ashamed to remove clothing with the light on, and may lead to being reluctant to be intimate with their partner. Negative body image can create barriers to communication and intimacy, ultimately impacting the quality of your sexual relationship.

Strategies for Boosting Self-Esteem and Body Image:

1. **Embrace Aging**: Recognize that aging is a natural part of life and focus on the positives that come with it, such as wisdom, experience, and personal growth. Cultivate a mindset of self-acceptance and gratitude for your body's resilience and capabilities.

2. **Practice Self-Compassion**: Be kind to yourself and challenge negative self-talk. Treat yourself with the same compassion and understanding that you would offer to a loved one facing similar struggles. Practice mindfulness and self-care to nurture emotional well-being.

3. **Stay Active**: Engage in regular physical activity to promote overall health and vitality. Exercise not only improves physical fitness but also boosts mood, self-confidence, and body image. Join a gym or put to use the exercise equipment that has been collecting dust in your garage or spare bedroom. Choose activities that you enjoy and that cater to your fitness level and abilities.

4. **Prioritize Intimacy**: Focus on the emotional connection and intimacy rather than solely on physical appearance or performance. Communicating openly with your partner about your desires, preferences, and your concerns about your body image, can foster trust, understanding, and mutual support.

5. **Explore Sensuality**: Rediscover pleasure and sensuality through sensual touch, massage, and other non-sexual activities. Take the time to explore each other's bodies and connect on a deeper level, savoring the moments of intimacy and closeness.

6. **Seek Support**: Don't hesitate to seek support from healthcare professionals, therapists, or a support group if you're struggling with self-esteem or body image issues. Professional guidance can provide valuable tools and strategies for coping with challenges and enhancing self-confidence.

Conclusion:

As we navigate the complexities of aging and intimacy, nurturing self-esteem and fostering a positive body image become essential pillars for maintaining a fulfilling happy sex life. By embracing your body, cultivating self-acceptance, and prioritizing intimacy, you can overcome barriers to sexual satisfaction and strengthen your emotional connection with your mate. Ultimately, a happy and healthy sex life in later years is not only possible but it is achievable. It can also enrich your overall well-being and the quality and longevity of your life.

Finding Support and Counseling

As we age, various aspects of life undergo transformations, including intimate relationships and sexual dynamics. Yet, the significance of maintaining a fulfilling sex life and intimacy doesn't diminish with age. For a senior couple, nurturing a healthy sexual relationship often requires dedicated support and at times counseling. Addressing physical changes, emotional needs, and relationship dynamics through professional guidance can profoundly enhance satisfaction and intimacy, fostering a vibrant and fulfilling connection for a happy sex life.

Understanding the Dynamics

As we have discussed throughout this guide, aging brings forth a myriad of changes, both physiological and psychological, that can impact sexual wellness. Physical factors such as hormonal shifts, chronic health conditions, and medication side effects can affect libido, arousal, and sexual function. Emotional changes, including stress, anxiety, and self-esteem issues, can also influence intimacy. Moreover, relational dynamics may evolve over time, necessitating adjustments in communication, connection, and sexual expression.

Breaking Stigma and Seeking Support

Despite the importance of sexual wellness in later life, as seniors, we often encounter societal taboos and ageist stereotypes that stigmatize discussions about sex and intimacy. Consequently, many of us may feel hesitant or ashamed to seek support or counseling for sexual concerns. However, breaking through these barriers and recognizing the value of professional assistance is crucial for promoting healthy sexual relationships and for developing a happy sex life. The benefits of counseling can address several of the concerns we have discussed throughout this guide:

Benefits of Counseling:

1. **Addressing Physical Challenges** - Professional counselors can offer insights into managing age-related physical changes that impact sexual function. From exploring alternative sexual activities to addressing concerns about erectile dysfunction or menopause-related

issues, counselors provide practical strategies for overcoming obstacles to intimacy.

2. **Navigating Emotional Barriers**: As seniors we may grapple with emotional barriers such as body image insecurities, past traumas, such as traumas from our childhood, or relationship conflicts that hinder sexual satisfaction. Counseling provides a safe space to explore these concerns, fostering emotional resilience and enhancing self-confidence.

3. **Improving Communication**: Effective communication lies at the heart of a fulfilling sexual relationship. A counselor can facilitate open and honest dialogues between you and your partner by encouraging both of you to express desires, concerns, and boundaries without judgment. Enhanced communication will foster greater intimacy and strengthen the bond between you and your mate.

4. **Rekindling Desire and Passion**: Through tailored interventions, a counselor can help reignite passion and desire within your relationship. From sensual exercises to mindfulness techniques, you and your mate can learn to reconnect on a deeper level, rediscovering intimacy and pleasure in your shared experiences.

5. **Supporting Relationship Dynamics**: As relationships evolve, conflicts and challenges may arise. Counseling can equip you and your mate with conflict-resolution skills, intimacy-building exercises, and strategies for sustaining emotional connection, thereby fostering resilience and an enduring partnership.

Conclusion:

Embracing sexual wellness in later life involves dispelling myths, challenging ageist stereotypes, and prioritizing open dialogue about intimacy and pleasure. By seeking support and counseling, you and your mate can navigate the complexities of aging while nurturing a fulfilling and satisfying sexual relationship. From overcoming physical challenges to deepening emotional intimacy, professional guidance can empower you and your partner to embrace your sexuality with confidence and joy, fostering a vibrant and enriching chapter in your lives.

Chapter 10: Exploring New Horizons

As we journey through life, the landscape of our desires and experiences evolves, and this holds true even for the realm of intimacy and sexuality, especially for us as senior citizens. Exploring new horizons in this aspect of life can be a transformative experience, vital for fostering a happy and fulfilling sex life.

For many of us, the idea of exploring new aspects of intimacy may seem daunting or even unnecessary. However, embracing novelty and adventure can breathe new life into a long-standing relationship, reigniting passion and deepening emotional connection. Here are several reasons why embracing new horizons is essential for maintaining a vibrant and satisfying sexual relationship in our senior years:

1. Combatting Routine:
Over time, sexual routines can develop within a relationship, leading to predictability and boredom. Breaking free from these patterns can invigorate intimacy, injecting excitement and spontaneity into the bedroom. A senior couple who actively seek out new experiences together can avoid falling into the trap of monotonous missionary position lovemaking, keeping their connection fresh and dynamic.

2. Rediscovering Pleasure:
As our bodies age, physical changes may occur that require adaptation and exploration. What once brought pleasure may no longer suffice, necessitating a journey of rediscovery. By experimenting with new techniques, positions, or forms of stimulation, you and your mate can uncover newfound sources of pleasure, enhancing your sexual satisfaction and intimacy.

3. Strengthening Communication:
As you, in the words of Mr. Spock, "live long and prosper", open and honest communication is the cornerstone of any healthy relationship, including sexual ones. Exploring new horizons will encourage you and your partner to communicate your desires, fantasies, and boundaries more effectively. Engaging in discussions about novel experiences fosters trust and intimacy, deepening the emotional connection between the two of you.

4. Fostering Connection:

Intimacy extends beyond physical acts; it encompasses emotional, intellectual, and spiritual connections as well. Exploring new horizons together allows you and your mate to bond on a deeper level, sharing adventures and creating cherished memories. Whether trying new activities, traveling to unfamiliar destinations, or learning new skills, shared experiences strengthen the foundation of the relationship, enriching both of your lives.

5. Embracing Growth:

Age should never be a barrier to personal growth and exploration. As you and your partner embrace new horizons, it demonstrates your willingness to evolve and adapt, both individually and as a couple. This mindset not only revitalizes your sex life but also promotes overall well-being and fulfillment as you continue to grow old gracefully together. Below are some practical tips for exploration:

1. **Educate Yourself:** Take advantage of resources such as books, workshops, videos, or online guides to learn about new techniques or sexual practices.

2. **Stay Open-Minded**: Approach new experiences with curiosity and a willingness to step outside your comfort zone.

3. **Prioritize Safety:** Always prioritize safety and consent when exploring new sexual activities or fantasies.

4. **Seek Professional Help**: If physical limitations or health concerns arise, consult with a healthcare professional or a sex therapist for guidance and support.

Conclusion:

The importance of exploring new horizons cannot be overstated when it comes to maintaining a happy and fulfilling sex life for you and your partner. By embracing novelty, fostering open communication, and prioritizing connection, the two of you can navigate the ever-changing landscape of intimacy with joy, passion, and mutual satisfaction. So, don't be afraid to embark together on this journey of discovery, for it is never too late to explore new frontiers of love and desire. This new adventure could cause your sexual relationship to, in Star Trex jargon, "boldly go where" it has "never gone before!"

Openness to New Experiences

As has been stated throughout this guide, sexuality is a fundamental aspect of human life that transcends age boundaries. However, as we grow older, societal perceptions often overshadow the importance of maintaining a fulfilling sex life in our senior years. Nevertheless, fostering openness to new experiences emerges as a crucial factor in revitalizing and enhancing the sexual relationship between you and your mate. In this section, we probe into the significance of openness to new experiences in rekindling passion, strengthening intimacy, and fostering renewed pleasure as you and your partner travel on this voyage to a happy sex life.

The Importance of Openness: Openness to new experiences encompasses a willingness to explore novel ideas, activities, and sensations. This trait holds immense significance in the context of senior sexuality as it breaks the barriers of routine and monotony, revitalizing the spark that may have diminished over the years. As a couple, embracing openness paves the way for rejuvenating your sexual relationship, thereby enhancing overall well-being and satisfaction.

Exploration and Discovery: One of the primary benefits of openness to new experiences in senior sexuality is the opportunity for exploration and discovery. As we age, we may become more set in our ways, leading to a sense of predictability in our sexual encounter. However, by fostering openness, you and your mate can embark on a journey of exploration, discovering new facets of intimacy and pleasure that you may not have previously explored. This sense of discovery injects excitement and novelty into your sex lives, reigniting passion and desire.

Communication and Connection: Openness also plays a pivotal role in fostering communication and connection between you and your partner. Effective communication is essential in expressing desires, preferences, and concerns, laying the foundation for a mutually satisfying sexual relationship. By embracing openness, you and your mate can engage in open and honest conversations about your sexual needs and desires, thus deepening your emotional bond and intimacy. This increased connection enhances trust and understanding, creating a supportive environment where both of you feel valued and heard.

Adaptability and Flexibility: As we age, changes in health, mobility, and physical abilities may necessitate adaptations in sexual practices. Openness to new experiences enables you to embrace these changes with flexibility and adaptability, rather than viewing them as obstacles. By being open to exploring alternative sexual activities, communication techniques, or intimacy-enhancing strategies, you and your mate can continue to enjoy fulfilling sexual experiences despite age-related challenges. This adaptability not only strengthens your sexual bond but also fosters resilience and acceptance in the face of change.

Embracing Sensuality: Openness to new experiences will encourage you and your partner to embrace sensuality in all its forms. This includes not only physical intimacy but also emotional, psychological, and spiritual connections. By expanding your definition of sexuality beyond conventional norms, the two of you can cultivate a deeper appreciation for sensual experiences such as kissing, caressing, fondling, and intimate conversation. This holistic approach to sensuality fosters a sense of fulfillment and satisfaction that transcends mere physical pleasure, enriching the overall quality of your sexual relationship.

Conclusion:
Openness to new experiences emerges as a cornerstone in nurturing a happy and fulfilling sex life for you and your partner. By embracing exploration, communication, adaptability, and sensuality, you and your mate can revitalize your sexual relationship, reigniting passion and intimacy in your golden years.

As society continues to evolve, it is essential to challenge ageist stereotypes and recognize the inherent value of sexuality as a senior citizen. Through openness and acceptance, your mate and you can embark on a journey of sexual fulfillment and joy, embracing the full spectrum of human intimacy regardless of age.

Sex Toys and Enhancements

We spoke extensively about sex toys and enhancements in chapter 7. In this chapter, we will reiterate the importance of considering these items to enhance your sexual repertoire. As society evolves, so do our perspectives on intimacy and sexual wellness. Through reading this guide, you now have a growing recognition of the importance of maintaining a fulfilling sex life well into older age. As a senior citizen couple, embracing sex toys and enhancements can be a transformative way to nurture intimacy, explore new sensations, and augment your sexual relationship.

Sex toys are items designed to enhance sexual pleasure and intimacy. They come in a variety of shapes, sizes, and functions, catering to different preferences and needs. Some common sex toys include: vibrators, dildos, anal toys, male masturbators, cock rings, and kegel balls. A specific description of each is presented in chapter 7.

Sexual Enhancements can include products like arousal gels, arousal oils, erection creams, or supplements designed to increase sexual desire, arousal, or performance. Sexual enhancements come in various forms, catering to different needs and preferences. Here are some common ones:

1. **Aphrodisiac Foods**: Certain foods like oysters, dark chocolate, strawberries, and watermelon are believed to enhance libido.

2. **Supplements**: There are numerous supplements on the market claiming to improve sexual performance and desire, such as L-arginine, L-citrulline, ginseng, and maca root.

3. **Medications**: Prescription medications like Viagra (sildenafil), Cialis (tadalafil), and Levitra (vardenafil) are commonly used to treat erectile dysfunction and can enhance sexual performance.

4. **Topical Products**: Gels, creams, and oils designed to increase sensitivity or arousal are available. Some contain ingredients like menthol or arginine.

5. **Erotic Literature and Media**: Reading erotica or watching erotic films can stimulate arousal and enhance sexual desire.

6. **Sex Talk**: Open communication, graphic sex talk, with your partner about desires, fantasies, and boundaries can enhance intimacy and sexual satisfaction.

7. **Yoga and Meditation**: Practices like yoga and meditation can help reduce stress and anxiety, which may improve sexual function and pleasure.

Please remember that not all enhancements work for everyone, and it's essential to consult with a healthcare professional before trying any new supplement or medication, especially if you have underlying health conditions or are taking other medications.

It's important to choose sex toys and enhancements that are made of body-safe materials, easy to clean, and suited to your preferences and comfort levels. Additionally, always communicate openly and honestly with your partner before introducing a sex toy into your sexual activities.

While the topic of sex toys and enhancements may still carry a degree of taboo, it's crucial to recognize that sexual desire and pleasure don't diminish with age. In fact, for many senior couples, the emotional and physical intimacy shared in their later years can be even more profound. However, as previously stated, factors such as menopause, erectile dysfunction, and other age-related changes can sometimes present challenges to sexual satisfaction. This is where sex toys and enhancements can play a vital role. Here are several reasons why sex toys and enhancements are particularly beneficial for senior couples:

Physical Changes: As we age, our bodies undergo various changes that can affect sexual function. As we discussed in greater detail in a previous chapter, for women, menopause can lead to vaginal dryness and decreased libido, while men may experience erectile difficulties or a decrease in sensitivity. Sex toys and enhancements, such as vibrators, lubricants, and arousal gels, can help address these issues by increasing comfort and pleasure during sexual activity.

Exploration and Variety: Long-term relationships can sometimes fall into a routine, leading to a decline in sexual excitement. Introducing sex toys and enhancements can inject novelty and excitement into the bedroom, encouraging couples to explore new sensations and experiences together. From vibrators and massage oils to bondage gear and role-playing costumes, to watching porn together, the possibilities are endless.

Enhanced Pleasure: Sex toys are designed to stimulate erogenous zones and intensify sensations, making sexual experiences more pleasurable for both partners. Whether used during foreplay or intercourse, toys like vibrating rings, dildos, and prostate massagers can enhance arousal and lead to more satisfying orgasms.

Communication and Connection: Introducing sex toys and enhancements into a relationship requires open communication and trust between you and your mate. Discussing preferences, desires, and boundaries can strengthen the emotional connection and deepen intimacy. Couples who explore these aspects of their relationship together often report feeling closer and more connected to each other.

Empowerment: Embracing sex toys and enhancements can empower you and your mate to take control of your sexual health and pleasure. Rather than viewing aging as a barrier to intimacy, you can see it as an opportunity to explore new avenues of pleasure and self-discovery. This sense of empowerment can have far-reaching effects, boosting confidence, self-esteem, and overall well-being.

It's important to note that there is no one-size-fits-all approach to sexual wellness, and what works for one couple may not work for another. Additionally, it's essential to prioritize safety, comfort, and mutual consent when using sex toys, especially for us older adults who may have underlying health conditions or emotional or spiritual apprehensions.

Conclusion:
Sex toys and enhancements can be invaluable tools in helping you and your mate to maintain a happy and fulfilling sex life. By embracing intimacy, exploring new experiences, and prioritizing communication, the two of you can continue to enjoy the physical and emotional benefits of sexual

connection throughout your life. As society continues to challenge stereotypes and taboos surrounding aging and sexuality, more senior couples are discovering that passion and pleasure can be achieved at any age.

Erotica and Sexual Fantasy

Erotica refers to literature, art, or other media that is designed to arouse sexual desire and excitement. It often focuses on explicit descriptions of sexual acts and situations, aiming to evoke sensual and passionate feelings in the audience. Unlike pornography, which primarily aims to depict sexual acts for the purpose of arousal, erotica often places more emphasis on the emotional and sensual aspects of sexual encounters and may explore themes such as desire, seduction, and intimacy in a more nuanced manner. As a genre, erotica can be found in various forms, including literature, films, photography, and visual art.

Sexual fantasy refers to imaginative thoughts or mental images that involve sexual scenarios, desires, or experiences. These fantasies can range from simple daydreams to elaborate narratives involving specific individuals, settings, or activities. They are a normal and common aspect of human sexuality.

Sexual fantasies can contribute to sexual arousal and can be used as a mental stimulant during sexual activities. Many sexual fantasies are private and may not necessarily reflect your mate's real-life desires or intentions. They provide a safe space for exploring and experimenting with sexual thoughts and scenarios.

In the realm of sexual intimacy, the vitality of erotica and sexual fantasy cannot be overstated. As you and your mate mature and embark on the journey of aging together, maintaining a fulfilling and happy sex life may pose unique challenges. However, embracing the power of erotica and sexual fantasy can be a transformative tool for reigniting passion and enhancing your sexual relationship.

Exploring Erotica: Erotica, with its rich narrative and sensual imagery, serves as a gateway to heightened arousal and exploration of desires. As a senior couple, delving into erotica offers an avenue to break free from the constraints of physical limitations and embrace the boundless realm of imagination. Whether through literature, film, or audio content, erotica provides a safe space for you and your partner to indulge in fantasies and reignite the flames of desire.

Importance of Sexual Fantasy: Sexual fantasy is the cornerstone of sexual exploration and fulfillment, regardless of age. As a senior citizen couple, nurturing a vibrant sexual fantasy life can inject excitement and novelty into your sexual relationship. Sexual fantasy allows both of you to transcend the limitations imposed by aging bodies and societal norms, enabling you to explore desires that may have remained dormant or unfulfilled.

Enhancing Intimacy: By incorporating erotica and sexual fantasy into your sex life, you and your mate can cultivate a deeper sense of intimacy and connection. Engaging in shared fantasies fosters open communication and trust, creating a safe environment for both of you to express your desires and vulnerabilities. Moreover, the exploration of sexual fantasies can reignite passion and desire, leading to greater satisfaction and fulfillment in the bedroom. For example, if you and your mate spent time reading an erotic novel, during intercourse, you both may be fantasizing that you were having sex with one of the characters you read about in the novel—and that's okay—as long as it is a part of your agreed upon fantasy activities.

Breaking Taboos: In many cultures, discussing sexuality and eroticism among older adults remains taboo. However, challenging these societal norms is essential for promoting sexual well-being and happiness. Embracing erotica and sexual fantasy empowers you and your partner to defy ageist stereotypes and reclaim your sexual agency. By embracing your desires and fantasies, your partner and you can forge a path toward greater sexual liberation and fulfillment.

Overcoming Challenges: While aging may bring physical changes that impact sexual function, it does not diminish the capacity for pleasure and intimacy. You may face challenges such as decreased libido, erectile dysfunction, or menopausal symptoms. However, by embracing erotica and sexual fantasy, you can navigate these obstacles with creativity and adaptability. Experimenting with new techniques, incorporating sensual erotica and sexual fantasy, or exploring alternative forms of pleasure can revitalize sexual intimacy and deepen the bond between you and your mate.

Conclusion:

In the journey of aging together, maintaining a happy and fulfilling sex life is a vital aspect of overall well-being and relationship satisfaction. By embracing erotica and sexual fantasy, you and your partner can transcend physical limitations, explore your desires, and reignite the flames of passion. Through open communication, trust, and a willingness to challenge societal taboos, your partner and you can embark on a journey of sexual exploration and rediscovery that brings joy, intimacy, and fulfillment to your lives.

Chapter 11: Single Seniors and Dating

If you are single, dating for a single senior citizen can be a wonderful and fulfilling experience. We all, regardless of age, are seeking companionship, love, and connection. This is especially true in our later years, and there are plenty of opportunities for us to find it. Remember, there's no age limit on love, and everyone deserves companionship and happiness even in the later years of life. So, embrace the dating journey and keep an open heart. This chapter provides some tips for you as you navigate the dating world.

Navigating Modern Dating

In today's fast-paced world, the dating landscape has undergone a significant transformation, with technology playing a pivotal role in connecting people of all ages. As a senior citizen, diving into the realm of modern dating might seem daunting at first, but with the right mindset and approach, it can be an enriching and fulfilling experience. Even if you have been out of the dating scene for a while, here are some tips to help you navigate modern dating with confidence:

1. **Stay Active**: Engage in activities and hobbies that you enjoy and that allow you to meet new people. This could be anything from joining a book club or a hiking group to taking a class or volunteering in your community. The more you put yourself out there, the higher your chances of meeting someone compatible.

2. **Embrace Technology (Try Online Dating)**: Embracing technology is essential in modern dating. Many seniors have found success in online dating. There are numerous dating websites and apps specifically designed for older adults, where you can connect with people who share your interests and values. A few of those websites have been listed in the Online Dating Tips of this chapter.

3. **Take Your Time**: There's no need to rush into anything. Take your time getting to know someone before committing to a relationship. Enjoy the process of getting to know each other and don't feel pressured to settle down quickly.

4. **Keep an Open Mind**: Be open to meeting people from diverse backgrounds and with different interests. You never know who you might click with! Don't dismiss someone based solely on age, appearance, or occupation. Give people a chance to surprise you. Keep an open mind when it comes to dating. You may meet someone who is different from what you expected but who ultimately makes you happy. Don't let age, race, religion, or any preconceived notions limit your potential for finding love.

5. **Pursue Your Passions**: Engaging in activities and hobbies you enjoy is not only fulfilling but also a great way to meet like-minded individuals. Join clubs, classes, or community events that align with your interests, whether it's dancing, painting, or hiking. You are more likely to meet a compatible partner when you share common passions.

6. **Be Patient**: Finding the right person takes time and patience. Don't get discouraged by setbacks or rejections. Stay positive and keep putting yourself out there. Remember that each date is an opportunity to learn and grow, regardless of the outcome.

7. **Communicate Effectively**: Effective communication is essential for building a strong and lasting relationship. Be clear and honest about your intentions, boundaries, and expectations from the start. Listen actively and empathetically to your dating partner's perspective, and don't be afraid to express your feelings openly.

8. **Communicate Honestly:** Be honest about your intentions and what you are looking for in a relationship. Communication is key, especially when it comes to discussing topics like past relationships, family, and future plans.

9. **Be Authentic:** Authenticity is important in building meaningful connections. Be honest about who you are, your interests, and what you are looking for in a partner. Don't feel pressured to conform to certain stereotypes or expectations. Be proud of your age and the wisdom and experiences it brings.

10. **Stay True to Yourself**: Always stay true to yourself and your values. Don't compromise your beliefs or interests for the sake of a relationship. The right person will appreciate you for who you are and embrace your uniqueness.

11. **Stay Safe**: Safety should always be a top priority when dating, especially online. Take precautions such as meeting in public places. Let a friend or family member know where you will be going and who you will be with, especially if you are meeting someone for the first time.

12. **Trust your Instincts**: Be wary of red flags such as requests for money or overly aggressive behavior. Trust your instincts and don't hesitate to leave a situation if you feel uncomfortable. Always prioritize your safety when dating.

13. **Have Fun:** Dating should be fun, regardless of your age. Approach it with a positive attitude and a sense of adventure. Even if you don't meet your soulmate right away, you will likely make new friends and create lasting memories along the way.

Conclusion:
Navigating modern dating as a senior citizen can be both exciting and challenging, but with the right mindset and approach, it can lead to fulfilling connections and companionship. By embracing technology, staying true to yourself, and keeping an open mind, you can embark on this journey with confidence and optimism. So go ahead, put yourself out there, and enjoy the adventure!

Online Dating Tips

In today's digital age, online dating has become a prevalent avenue for people of all ages to find companionship, love, and meaningful connections. While the prospect of diving into the world of online dating may seem daunting for you as a senior citizen, it can also be an exciting opportunity to meet new people and explore romantic possibilities. With the right approach and mindset, you can navigate online dating platforms with confidence and success. Here are some valuable tips to help you make the most of your online dating experience:

Choose the Right Platform: With numerous online dating websites and apps available, it's essential to select a platform that caters to your specific interests and preferences. Some platforms are designed for casual dating, while others focus on long-term relationships. Take the time to research different options and choose one that aligns with your goals. Familiarize yourself with popular dating apps and websites tailored for seniors, such as *OurTime*, *SilverSingles*, or *SeniorMatch*. These platforms offer a comfortable and convenient way to meet like-minded individuals in your age group.

Create an Honest Profile: When creating your online dating profile, honesty is key. Be truthful about your age, interests, and intentions. Use recent photos that accurately represent yourself, and write a bio that reflects your personality and what you are looking for in a partner.

Take it Slow: In the age of instant gratification, it's important to take things slow and not rush into anything. Get to know your potential matches gradually through messaging or phone calls. This allows you to gauge compatibility and establish a rapport before taking the next step.

Take Your Time: Don't feel pressured to rush into anything. Take your time getting to know someone before agreeing to meet in person. Engage in meaningful conversations, ask questions, and look for common interests. Building a connection online can take time, so be patient and enjoy the process.

Be Open-Minded: Keep an open mind when interacting with potential matches. Don't dismiss someone based solely on age or other superficial factors. Be willing to explore different connections and give people a chance to surprise you.

Stay Positive: Online dating can sometimes feel overwhelming or discouraging, especially if you don't immediately find a compatible match. Stay positive and maintain a hopeful outlook. Remember that the right person is out there, and each interaction brings you one step closer to finding them.

Be Yourself: Authenticity is attractive, so be yourself throughout the online dating journey. Don't try to portray a false image or pretend to be someone you are not. Embrace your unique qualities and let your personality shine.

Have Realistic Expectations: While online dating can lead to fulfilling relationships, it's essential to have realistic expectations. Not every interaction will result in a love connection, and that's okay. Approach each interaction as an opportunity to learn and grow.

Stay Safe: Safety should always be a top priority when engaging in online dating. Be cautious about sharing personal information such as your home address, phone number, or financial details. Use the platform's messaging system to communicate initially, and only meet in person when you feel comfortable and ready. When personally meeting a person you met online, always meet in public places—preferably during the day. Be sure to inform a friend or family member of your location.

Enjoy the Journey: Above all, remember to have fun and enjoy the journey of online dating. Treat it as an adventure filled with new experiences and possibilities. Stay true to yourself, stay safe, and remain open to the exciting opportunities that online dating can bring.

Stay Open to Offline Opportunities: While online dating is a convenient way to meet people, don't overlook offline opportunities to socialize and meet potential partners. Attend church, community events, join clubs or groups, and engage in activities that interest you. You never know where you might meet someone special.

Conclusion:
Online dating can be a rewarding experience, offering a chance to connect with like-minded individuals and potentially find love later in life. By following the tips given in this section and approaching the process with an open heart and mind, you can navigate the world of digital romance with confidence and optimism.

Building A New Relationship

Entering the world of dating and romance after a divorce or the loss of a spouse can be a daunting prospect at any age. However, for senior citizens, the idea of starting over can feel particularly overwhelming. Yet, despite the challenges, many seniors find themselves longing for companionship and the warmth of a new romantic relationship. In this section, we explore how you can navigate this journey with courage, optimism, and resilience.

Embrace Self-Discovery: The first step in building a new romantic relationship as a senior citizen is to embark on a journey of self-discovery. Take the time to reflect on your values, interests, and aspirations. What are the qualities you seek in a partner? What brings you joy and fulfillment? By gaining a deeper understanding of yourself, you will be better equipped to attract a compatible partner who shares your values and interests.

Cultivate Social Connections: Building a new romantic relationship often begins with expanding your social circle. Engage in activities and hobbies that you enjoy, whether it's joining a book club, a gym, the local senior citizen center, taking a dance class, or volunteering in your community. These opportunities not only allow you to meet new people but also provide a platform for meaningful interactions and connections.

Be Open-Minded: It's important to approach the dating process with an open mind and heart. Be willing to step outside your comfort zone and explore new possibilities. Keep in mind that everyone comes with their own unique background and experiences. Embrace the opportunity to learn from each other and appreciate the differences that make each individual special.

Take Things Slowly: Rushing into a new relationship after a divorce or loss of a spouse can be tempting, but it's essential to take things slowly and allow the relationship to develop organically. Take the time to get to know each other on a deeper level, building trust and emotional intimacy along the way. Enjoy the journey of discovery and savor each moment spent together.

Communicate Effectively: Communication is key in any relationship, especially when starting anew. Be open and honest with your partner about your feelings, expectations, and concerns. Listen attentively to their thoughts and emotions, and strive to find common ground. Effective communication lays the foundation for a strong and healthy relationship built on mutual respect and understanding.

Seek Support: Navigating the complexities of romance and relationships can be challenging, especially after a significant life transition. Don't hesitate to seek support from friends, family members, a clergy, or a professional counselor who can offer guidance and encouragement along the way. Surround yourself with a supportive network of people who uplift and empower you on your journey to finding love again.

Building a New Sexual Relationships After Divorce or Death of a Spouse

In a society where discussions about sexuality often revolve around youth and vitality, the topic of sexual relationships among senior citizens can sometimes be overlooked or even taboo. However, the reality is that many seniors desire and enjoy intimacy well into their later years. Whether due to divorce or the loss of a spouse, entering into a new sexual relationship as a senior citizen can present unique challenges and opportunities. Let's explore how in this stage of life you can navigate this aspect of a new relationship with care and confidence.

Embracing Change and Growth: The end of a marriage, whether through divorce or death, marks a significant transition in one's life. It's natural to experience a range of emotions during this time, including grief, loneliness, and even a sense of liberation. However, it's essential to recognize that life doesn't end with the dissolution of a relationship. Instead, it opens up new possibilities for personal growth and fulfillment, including the potential for intimate connections with another.

Self-Exploration and Reflection: Before embarking on a new sexual relationship, it's crucial for you to engage in self-exploration and reflection. This involves taking the time to understand your own desires, boundaries, and expectations regarding intimacy. What are your values and beliefs about sex and relationships? What do you hope to gain from a sexual partnership at this stage of your life? Being clear about these aspects can help guide you in making decisions that align with your needs and preferences.

Communication and Consent: Open and honest communication is key to any successful relationship, and this holds especially true before entering a new sexual relationship. It's essential to have candid conversations with the potential partner about your intentions, desires, and any concerns or boundaries you may have. Likewise, it's important to actively listen to your partner's perspective and be respectful of their needs and boundaries.

Moreover, consent remains paramount at all stages of a sexual relationship, regardless of age. Both parties should feel comfortable expressing their consent or lack thereof, and any sexual activity should be mutually agreed upon and enjoyable for both individuals.

Exploring New Horizons: Entering into a new sexual relationship as a senior citizen can be an opportunity to explore new horizons and rediscover aspects of yourself. This may involve trying new activities or experiences in the bedroom, as well as cultivating emotional intimacy and connection with your partner. It's important to approach these experiences with an open mind and a sense of curiosity, allowing yourself to embrace pleasure and fulfillment in whatever form it may take.

Seeking Support and Resources: Navigating the complexities of a sexual relationship as a senior citizen may sometimes require external support and resources. This could involve seeking guidance from a therapist or counselor who specializes in issues related to sexuality and aging. Additionally, there are numerous books, workshops, and online communities dedicated to helping seniors explore intimacy and relationships in later life.

Conclusion:
Building a new romantic relationship as a senior citizen after divorce or the death of a spouse is a journey filled with both challenges and opportunities. By embracing self-discovery, cultivating social connections, and maintaining an open mind and heart, you can embark on this journey with courage and optimism. While the prospect of building a sexual relationship after divorce or the death of a spouse may seem daunting, it's important to remember that love, desire, and intimacy are not limited by age. You have every right to pursue a fulfilling sexual relationship that brings joy and companionship into your life. By embracing change, communicating openly, and exploring new horizons, you can cultivate meaningful connections that enhance your overall well-being and quality of life. With patience, communication, and support,

love has the power to flourish once again, bringing joy, companionship, and fulfillment in its wake.

Chapter 12: Resources and Support

In the realm of relationships, intimacy is a cornerstone that evolves and adapts over time. For a senior citizen couple, nurturing a fulfilling and satisfying sex life is not only possible but also crucial for overall well-being. However, this journey may come with its unique set of challenges. Fortunately, with the right resources and support, you and your partner can navigate these challenges and cultivate a vibrant and happy sex life.

Understanding the Challenges: We have discussed throughout this guide that aging brings about various physiological and psychological changes that can impact sexual health and intimacy. Hormonal shifts, chronic health conditions, and medication side effects are just a few factors that may affect sexual desire, function, and satisfaction in older adults. We have also discussed the fact that societal attitudes and misconceptions about aging and sexuality can contribute to our feelings of shame, embarrassment, or inadequacy. However, having the proper resources and support can help to alleviate these challenges.

Throughout this guide, we have in one form or another discussed the importance of resources and support. Through our discussions on educational materials, support networks, communication, and emotional connection, exploring alternative means of intimacy, and embracing adaptation—we have highlighted the importance of resources and support for having a happy sex life in your senior years. Below is a recap of some of the topics we have discussed:

Resources: Access to accurate information and resources is fundamental for a senior couple seeking to enhance their sexual relationship. Educational materials, workshops, and online resources can provide valuable insights into age-related changes in sexuality, techniques for maintaining sexual health, and strategies for overcoming common obstacles. Additionally, healthcare professionals specializing in geriatric care can offer personalized advice and guidance tailored to individual needs.

Support Networks: We have shared with you on several occasions in this guide the fact that navigating the complexities of aging and intimacy may feel overwhelming for a senior couple. This is where support networks play a crucial role. Peer support groups, whether in-person or online, offer a safe space for you and your mate to share experiences, seek advice, and offer encouragement. Connecting with others who are facing similar challenges can foster a sense of solidarity and empowerment, alleviating feelings of isolation and stigma.

Communication and Emotional Connection: Throughout this guide, we have pointed out that effective communication is the cornerstone of any healthy relationship, especially when it comes to intimacy. You and your mate are encouraged to openly discuss your desires, concerns, and boundaries with each other. By fostering honest and respectful communication, you and your partner can deepen your emotional connection and build trust, laying the foundation for a fulfilling sex life.

Exploring Alternative Intimacy: As has been stated on numerous occasions in this guide, intimacy encompasses a broad spectrum of physical and emotional connections beyond sexual activity. You and your mate throughout this guide have been encouraged to explore alternative forms of intimacy, such as cuddling, kissing, and sensual touching. These acts of affection can foster intimacy and closeness, regardless of any physical limitations or challenges.

Embracing Adaptation: You have also been encouraged through the pages of this guide that in order to rejuvenate your sex life, you and your mate should embrace a mindset of adaptation and flexibility. This may involve adjusting expectations, exploring new sexual techniques, taking more time during foreplay, or incorporating assistive sexual devices to enhance pleasure and comfort. By embracing change and being open to experimentation, your partner and you can discover new avenues for intimacy and satisfaction.

Conclusion:
A happy and fulfilling sex life is not exclusive to youth; it's a journey that continues to evolve and flourish throughout the lifespan. Leveraging resources and support is essential in navigating the complexities of aging and intimacy. By accessing accurate information, fostering open communication, and embracing adaptation, you and your mate can cultivate a vibrant,

fulfilling, and happy sexual relationship that enhances your overall well-being and quality of life for as long as you both shall live.

Professional Help and Counseling

Here's a list of professional help and counseling organizations that work to improve the sexual relationship of senior citizen couples:

1. **American Association of Sexuality Educators, Counselors, and Therapists (AASECT)**: AASECT provides certification for professionals specializing in sexuality education, counseling, and therapy. They have a directory of certified therapists who may work with senior couples.

2. **American Psychological Association (APA)**: APA has a directory of psychologists who specialize in various areas, including sex therapy and relationship counseling. Senior couples may find suitable therapists through this directory.

3. **National Council on Aging (NCOA)**: NCOA offers various resources for older adults, including information on sexual health and relationships in later life. They may provide referrals to counselors or therapists who specialize in working with seniors.

4. **Sexuality and Aging Consortium at Widener University**: This consortium focuses on promoting research, education, and advocacy on sexuality and aging. They may have resources or referrals for senior couples seeking counseling.

5. **National Sexuality Resource Center (NSRC)**: NSRC provides resources and training on sexuality-related topics, including aging and sexuality. They may have information on counselors or therapists who specialize in this area.

6. **Society for Sex Therapy and Research (SSTAR)**: SSTAR is an organization of professionals dedicated to the advancement of knowledge in the field of sex therapy and research. They may have a directory of therapists who work with older adults.

7. **Local Aging Services Organizations**: Many local organizations focused on aging and senior services may offer counseling or support groups for older adults on various topics, including sexuality and relationships.

8. **Geriatric Social Workers or Counselors**: Geriatric social workers or counselors specializing in aging issues may offer counseling services for senior couples, including addressing sexual concerns.

9. **University Affiliated Counseling Centers**: Many universities with counseling psychology or social work programs may offer counseling services to the community. They may have therapists who specialize in working with older adults.

10. **Senior Centers or Community Centers**: Some senior centers or community centers may offer workshops, support groups, or counseling services specifically geared towards addressing sexual health and relationships in later life.

When seeking help, it's essential that you find professionals who are knowledgeable and experienced in working with your specific needs and concerns related to sexual intimacy in later life.

Books, Websites, and Community Groups

Here's a list of resources that can help senior citizen couples improve their sexual relationship:

Books:

1. "Better Than I Ever Expected: Straight Talk about Sex After Sixty" by Joan Price

2. "The Ultimate Guide to Sex After Fifty: How to Maintain – or Regain – a Spicy, Satisfying Sex Life" by Joan Price

3. "Naked at Our Age: Talking Out Loud About Senior Sex" by Joan Price

4. "Sex Over 50: Updated and Expanded" by Joel D. Block and Kimberly Dawn Neumann

5. "The Joy of Sex: The Ultimate Revised Edition" by Alex Comfort and Susan Quilliam

Websites:

1. **Senior Sex Matters**: A website offering articles, resources, and advice specifically tailored to older adults' sexual health and relationships. (seniorsexmatters.com)

2. **AARP**: AARP provides information and resources on a wide range of topics for seniors, including sexual health and relationships. (aarp.org)

3. **Everyday Health (Senior Health)**: Everyday Health has a dedicated section on senior health, including articles on sexual health and intimacy for older adults. (everydayhealth.com/senior-health)

4. **Sexual Health for Older Adults – Planned Parenthood**: Planned Parenthood offers information and resources on sexual health for people of all ages, including seniors. (plannedparenthood.org/learn/sexual-health-older-adults)

5. **Senior Planet**: Senior Planet is a website and community for older adults covering various topics, including relationships and sexuality. (seniorplanet.org)

Community Groups:

1. **Local Senior Centers**: Many local senior centers organize workshops, support groups, and events focused on various aspects of senior life, including relationships and sexuality.

2. **Meetup**: This online platform is where seniors can find local groups and events related to their interests, including those focused on improving sexual relationships (meetup.com).

3. **Senior-Specific Dating Sites**: While primarily for dating, some senior-specific dating sites may also have forums or community

sections where members can discuss topics related to relationships and sexuality with peers.

4. **Healthcare Provider Support Groups**: Some healthcare providers, especially those specializing in geriatric care or sexual health, may organize support groups or workshops for older adults.

5. **Online Forums and Discussion Boards**: There are online forums and discussion boards specifically dedicated to topics related to senior sexuality and relationships where individuals can seek advice and support from peers.

These resources can provide valuable information, support, and guidance as you seek to improve your sexual relationship and overall intimacy.

Continuing Education on Sexual Health

Here's a list of continuing education programs and resources that focus on improving the sexual relationship of senior citizen couples:

1. **American Association of Sexuality Educators, Counselors, and Therapists (AASECT)**: AASECT offers various workshops, webinars, and certification programs for professionals working in the field of sexual health and therapy. Some of these may cover topics related to senior sexuality.

2. **International Society for Sexual Medicine (ISSM)**: ISSM provides educational resources, conferences, and webinars focusing on sexual medicine, including issues related to sexual health in older adults.

3. **American Society on Aging (ASA)**: ASA offers resources, webinars, and conferences on aging-related topics, including sexuality in older adults.

4. **Sexual Health and Aging: A Continuing Education Program for Nurses (University of California, San Francisco)**: This online course focuses on understanding sexual health issues in older adults

and providing appropriate care. It covers topics such as sexual function, intimacy, and communication.

5. **National Association of Social Workers (NASW)**: NASW offers continuing education opportunities for social workers, some of which may cover topics related to sexual health and relationships in older adults.

6. **The American Academy of Nurse Practitioners (AANP)**: AANP provides educational resources and conferences for nurse practitioners, some of which may address sexual health concerns in older adults.

7. **Society for Sex Therapy and Research (SSTAR)**: SSTAR offers conferences, workshops, and resources for professionals in the field of sex therapy and research, which may include content on senior sexuality.

8. **American Counseling Association (ACA)**: ACA offers continuing education opportunities for counselors, including courses or workshops that focus on sexual health and intimacy in older adults.

9. **Sexual Medicine Society of North America (SMSNA)**: SMSNA provides educational resources and conferences focusing on sexual medicine, which may include discussions on sexual health in older adults.

10. **The American Association of Nurse Practitioners (AANP)**: AANP offers educational resources and conferences for nurse practitioners, some of which may address sexual health concerns in older adults.

These resources can provide valuable information and strategies as you work to improve your sexual relationship. It's essential to check the specific offerings of each organization to ensure they align with your needs and interests.

In closing, *A Senior Citizen Guide to a Happy Sex Life* is not just a guide; it's a celebration of vitality, intimacy, and the enduring power of love at any age. As you navigate the golden years, may these pages serve as a reminder that passion knows no bounds, and with understanding, communication, and a willingness to embrace change, the journey of sexual fulfillment can be one of joy, connection, and endless discovery.

Here's to embracing the full spectrum of life's pleasures, regardless of the number of candles on your birthday cake. Cheers to love, laughter, and a happy, fulfilling sex life for you and your mate, now and forever!

Made in the USA
Columbia, SC
10 July 2024

38440236R00074